# FEAR Made You Fat & Not Calories

## Just 4 Steps to End the Obesity Epidemic

Ronald Fisher, ND

Caryn Wichmann, ND

ISBN-10: 1466390697
ISBN-13: 978-1466390690

# DEDICATION

We dedicate this work to our many clients who have participated in testing our weight loss methods and who have made an incredible contribution to this work by their valued feedback and enthusiasm.

# CONTENTS

Acknowledgements    i

1  Introduction    1

2  FEAR Made You Fat    4

3  Fructose in Everything – Its Part in the Obesity Epidemic    6

4  Exercise Reduction – Its Part in the Obesity Epidemic    13

5  Artificial Trans Fat – Its Part in the Obesity Epidemic    19

6  Reduced Key Nutrients – Its Part in the Obesity Epidemic    26

7  Gaining Control of Your Life    36

8  Turn Disease into Good Health    46

9  Don't Buy It & Watch Your Finances Improve    57

10  How to Turn McDonalds into McHealthy    61

11  A People's Health Revolution    63

# ACKNOWLEDGMENTS

The researchers and technical support staff at Bioconcepts Australia and Metagenics Australia have been incredibly supportive in our quest for the underlying causes of weight gain.

Our work would not have been possible without the many groups of dedicated researchers around the world who regularly publish their findings in free access format on the internet.

Although confidentiality prevents us from listing the names of our clients, we cannot understate the invaluable contribution they have made in monitoring their symptoms and reporting the effectiveness of various treatment options. The discovery that any of the four elements of FEAR can actually combine to keep anyone in 'fat storage mode' came directly from analyzing the feedback of our clients. Clients attending our clinic on a regular basis for measurements and other assessments was essential for our work and we cannot thank them enough for the their regular attendance. The body of knowledge that we have developed around weight gain and weight loss is largely attributable to the dedication of our clients.

# 1   INTRODUCTION

In our clinic we see overweight and obese people on a daily basis.  In fact the number of overweight and obese people is at epidemic proportions.   Our success rate at treating this condition was acceptable by industry standards with around 80% of clients losing weight and improving their health considerably with the remaining 20% gaining some improvement but not enough to be regarded as healthy.   This 20% worried us and made us constantly research for more solutions.  Another worrying issue was that many patients could not lose that last 5 to 10 kilograms of fat mainly around the abdominal area but sometimes around hips and thighs.  We also had clients who were not overweight by medical standards but still had unwanted fat accumulating, particularly around the abdomen.

Researchers at the University of Pennsylvania School of Medicine[1] made an important finding that although much attention has been focused on diet and exercise, these strategies alone are not effective at solving the world wide health crisis.  The worldwide health crisis is a big issue.  World Health Organisation estimates showed that in 2008, 1.5 billion adults aged 20 years and older were overweight and over 200 million men and 300 million women — approximately 10% of adults — were obese worldwide.  Other research shows that weight gain is just as big a problem with children.   Obesity is no longer a problem for high-income developed countries alone.  Since 1980 large increases in obesity have occurred in low and middle-income countries, particularly in urban settings in Oceania, Latin America, and North Africa.  The spread of obesity follows the spread of the "Western Diet" and people who stay with indigenous diets rich in vegetables, fruits, and fish usually do not suffer the epidemic.  Because diet and exercise alone does not appear to solve the epidemic the researchers recommended that a more in depth look at the biochemistry of what was happening was needed.  When you also consider the problem that fat accumulation also extends to people who are not technically overweight, it seemed obvious that the issue that we were looking for is widespread and virtually affects everybody.

It was clear that calorie counting alone combined with exercise, although having some benefits does not solve the problem and that other issues are involved that affected most people and was preventing satisfactory weight loss and was probably responsible for weight gain.

Anybody who has struggled to achieve something in their life knows how important it is to be healthy and even more importantly, to look healthy, vibrant and energetic to other people. Being healthy is much more than being free of symptoms of disease. It is all about having the energy and physical fitness to enjoy all the opportunities and challenges that occur in the world around us, and to make the most of our lives. When you achieve this level of good health, you have the energy and enthusiasm to turn the negatives into positives, to do constructive work, to maintain friendships, to be part of a family, to participate in sports, to travel, to enjoy nature, to create wealth for yourself and others around you, to help others and to do all the great things that are on offer. When you are in this level of good health you can eat a variety of healthy foods and you do not gain weight. There appeared to be something that was stopping people achieving this level of vitality.

Interpreting scientific evidence and using this knowledge to provide practical and useable health improvement solutions for our clients had always been a major focus for us. We decided to allocate much more time to research and to testing alternative solutions to the weight loss problem. The results of this work prompted us to write this book.

Apart from gaining weight there are many warning signs and symptoms that indicate your health is deteriorating. These signs and symptoms included being irritable, anxious, having low energy, moody, lacking sleep, experiencing recurring pain, procrastination, nail biting, nausea, jaw clenching, poor concentration, infertility, sexual dysfunction, agitation, ulcers, overdoing activities, backache, skin problems, depressive episodes, rashes, constant worrying, hair loss, diarrhoea, constipation, general unhappiness, unable to build muscle, cold sores, allergies, etc, etc. Even having one of these issues is significant and should not be ignored. Many people ignore these signs and symptoms of poor health, and even medically trained clinicians will often ignore them to their own detriment. Ignoring these early warning signs results in compensatory action within your body which eventually leads to more serious health conditions like depression, obesity, cardiovascular disease, cancer, allergies, autoimmune diseases, arthritis, wrinkled and 'old looking' skin, etc. The biochemistry behind each of these signs and symptoms is quite complex and when analysed thoroughly can lead to different treatment plans for each person. However, even when a client followed their individually designed treatment plan there was no guarantee that they would lose all the unwanted fat, or achieve the ultimate levels of good health that we aim for.

We wanted answers and so we devoted the time to analysing our client results and reviewing research until we had a simple practical solution.

The answer was that FEAR makes you fat and reversing it is the road to weight loss and good health.

## References

1.    Ahima RS, 2011, Digging deeper into obesity, Journal of Clinical Investigation, 121(6):2076–2079, doi:10.1172/JCI58719

# 2 FEAR MADE YOU FAT

The word FEAR has two meanings in regard to weight gain and the obesity epidemic.

The first meaning is that FEAR stands for:

F = Fructose in everything

E = Exercise reduction

A = Artificial Trans Fats

R = Reduced key nutrients

Over the last 50 years or so our "modern" industrialised society has inflicted these four elements of FEAR onto its citizens in frightening proportions. In the following chapters we will explain each one of these issues with a summary of the facts, the details of the research that demonstrates the dimensions of the issue and the specific actions you can take to overcome each issue. It is important to recognise that each one of these four elements of FEAR work together to cause the obesity epidemic and just solving one does not solve the problem – all the issues need to be addressed – the combined effect is more important than any individual component.

The second meaning of FEAR refers to people within organisations who fear change. As the scientific evidence slowly accumulated showing the depth of the problem with processed foods, sweetened drinks and junk food combinations the massive resources of the organisations involved were devoted to preventing change by lobbying politicians, increasing advertising or creating conflicting arguments rather than simply addressing the issues. In our chapter on "Don't Buy It" we aim to address this aspect of fear and demonstrate that changes can be made without destroying the jobs of thousands of people or closing down major enterprises. Just to prove how easily the world could be changed into an incredibly healthy place, we have provided a chapter on what most people would regard as impossible - "How to turn a McDonalds restaurant into a place that supports good health in four simple steps – we call this new restaurant McHealthy".

It is common that overweight and obese people believe that they do not have the will power to make significant changes to their lives. These people are often lonely, stressed and possibly depressed. We have devoted a chapter to demonstrating that there are some simple practical ways to gain control of your life and help with the reversal of FEAR.

Many people have been exposed to the elements of FEAR for long periods and are now in a state of chronic disease. We have devoted a chapter of the book to demonstrating how you can turn a disease state into a good health state.

The four steps needed to reverse the FEAR generated obesity epidemic are easy to understand and easy to implement. All you need to do is decide to do it. The final chapter in our book describes how you can apply FEAR reversal to yourself and how you can spread the message to the 2 billion plus people throughout the world who need to know that FEAR made you fat.

# 3 FRUCTOSE IN EVERYTHING – ITS PART IN THE OBESITY EPIDEMIC

**Summary**

The main point that we want you to take away from this chapter is that consuming significant amounts of fructose at the same time as other foods (i.e. fats, carbohydrates and protein) puts you into fat storage mode. So the fructose doesn't actually make you fat it just tells your body to store most of the other food that you are currently digesting as fat. This combination effect goes beyond the other foods you are eating. It extends to the signals that are also being received about muscles, heart, brain, bone, etc which regulates what will be needed to be stored – the other elements of FEAR stimulate you to store even more as fat.

Thus not consuming fructose at the same time as other foods is just step one in the process of losing weight. You have to implement all the elements of FEAR reversal. So don't expect miracles because you have been good and moved your fructose consumption to well away from other foods, it will only help you if you implement the other 3 elements of FEAR reversal.

**Now let's look at what we know about fructose and how we know it**

The evidence that fructose was a major issue in weight gain has been accumulating for some time. Some researchers[1,2,3] believed that the increasing consumption of sweetened drinks was directly linked to the obesity epidemic. These and other researchers[4] were highlighting the role of fructose in sweetened drinks, particularly the role of High Fructose Corn Syrup which was widely used by the food industry, and linking this with obesity and disease. One study[5] linked fructose in sweetened drinks (and not glucose) to general weight gain as well as specific abdominal weight gain. However, the specific mechanism by which fructose stimulated weight gain was not clear and the food industry was extremely reluctant to give up this cheap form of sweetener. We, like most other practitioners in the weight loss industry, advised our clients to avoid sweetened drinks and most clients confirmed it supported their weight loss efforts. What wasn't clear is whether we were just cutting calories or whether the removal of sweetened drinks had other benefits.

At the time of writing this book the best summary available of the specific action of fructose in relation to weight gain is provided in a review article[6] prepared by researchers at the Division of Renal Diseases and Hypertension at the University of Colorado Denver in collaboration with researchers at the Nicolaus Copernicus University in Toru´n, Poland and published in June 2011. The researchers stated that a review of all the evidence was convincing that an excessive intake of fructose had an etiologic role in the epidemic of obesity, diabetes, and cardiorenal disease. The more important issue for us was the biochemical mechanism where fructose consumption effectively put your body into fat storage mode was a compelling argument for the role of fructose. This meant that anyone wanting to lose weight could not afford to consume any significant amounts of fructose at the same time as other foods because they would not be able to lose weight while they were in fat storage mode. When you link this knowledge with the other three aspects of FEAR you start to appreciate how easily the obesity epidemic came about and how simple it would be to reverse it.

The researchers explain that fructose is absorbed into the intestine enterocyte by the Glut-5 specific transporter. While some fructose is metabolized in the small intestinal wall, much of it is passed via the portal vein to the liver, with perhaps 20 to 30% escaping into the systemic circulation. Within the hepatocyte, fructose is phosphorylated to fructose-1-phosphate by fructokinase. Because this reaction has no negative feedback system, if sufficient fructose is present, intracellular phosphate and ATP depletion can transiently occur. This results in the generation of AMP which is metabolized by AMP deaminase to inosine monophosphate and eventually to uric acid. The transient ATP depletion has some similarities to ischemia and can result in arrest of protein synthesis with the induction of oxidative stress and inflammation.

Now if fructose was just consumed by itself with a moderate amount of carbohydrate present (as in a piece of fruit) then none of this mechanism would trigger weight gain. Natural fruits also are rich in antioxidants, ascorbate, polyphenols, potassium, and fibre that may counter the effects of fructose. The issue is firstly, the presence of significant amounts of fats, carbohydrates and proteins at the same time that fructose is going through this process in the liver and secondly, whether you repeatedly expose your body to this process over a long period of time. Fructose is known to stimulate fat accumulation in the liver by both increasing synthesis and blocking fat oxidation[7]. Fructose is also known to stimulate glycogen accumulation in the liver [8,9] which appears to be due to inhibiting glycogenolysis due to inhibition of glycogen phosphorylase[10]. We also know that chronically high consumption of fructose in rodents leads to hepatic and extrahepatic insulin resistance, obesity, type 2 diabetes mellitus, and high blood pressure[11]. Fructose overconsumption has also been shown to cause dyslipidemia (abnormal amount of lipids such as cholesterol or fat in the blood) and ectopic lipid deposition in healthy subjects with and without a family history of type 2 diabetes[12]. So over a period of time the combination of significant amounts of fructose with other foods (particularly fats and carbohydrates) puts you into a state of fat accumulation, generating high levels of energy becomes harder to achieve and weight loss becomes increasingly difficult.

Remember that it is FEAR that made you fat and not just fructose. So not only does fructose act in combination with the other foods that you consumed at the same time, fructose also acts in combination with "E" exercise reduction, "A" artificial trans fats and "R" reduced key nutrients. Reduced exercise signals that energy should be stored as fat instead of replacing glycogen stores. Artificial trans fats can reduce the capacity of the liver even if it is some time ago that you consumed your last trans fat. Being deficient in a few key nutrients can also signal that you should remain in fat storage mode or possibly reduce the rate at which you burn energy. As an example reduced vitamin D can reduce your metabolism rate and if other nutrients like vitamin K, magnesium, calcium and proteins are low, then your body will not be rebuilding bone and muscle and be signalling that energy is not needed for these purposes and to stay in fat storage mode. So when debating the actual biochemical mechanics of fructose it is important to remember that more than one thing is going on in your body and a combination of factors needs to be considered.

If there were only very small quantities of fructose in the diet the biochemical mechanism would only be temporarily in this mode but with the large amount of fructose found in the modern western diet the result is item number one in the FEAR generated obesity epidemic.

Another issue with consuming any form of sugar in quantity is that the end result is a high level of glucose in the blood which must be managed by various mechanisms but mainly by insulin. Constantly demanding that your body generate high insulin levels will obviously cause some type of problem in the long run – your pancreas just wasn't designed to constantly pump out high amounts of insulin. The other important functions of the pancreas such as production of pancreatic enzymes may be compromised simply because the pancreas has too much of its resources allocated to insulin production.

Before we look at what you can do about fructose we need to look at the condition called 'Insulin Resistance'.

Insulin resistance is a condition where insulin (a natural hormone) becomes less effective at lowering blood sugars. The resulting increase in blood glucose may raise levels outside the normal range and cause adverse health effects. Certain cell types such as fat and muscle cells require insulin to absorb glucose. When these cells fail to respond adequately to circulating insulin, blood glucose levels rise. The liver helps to regulate glucose levels by reducing its secretion of glucose in the presence of insulin. This normal reduction in the liver's glucose production may not occur in people with insulin resistance. So people with unmanaged insulin resistance may not be able to deposit glucose in fat cells when they need to and they may not be able to take it out when they need to.

Thus the process of insulin regulation means that not everybody will experience insulin resistance to the same degree or have the same consequences. With some of our weight loss clients we find that they are living on a diet that just keeps them sustained and they can't lose weight because the available mechanisms to remove fat from fat cells including the needed levels of insulin are not working properly.

Thus in addition to reversing FEAR some people may need to seek out a health practitioner who can prescribe a treatment for insulin resistance or some other related condition. There is more about this issue in our chapter on 'Turning Disease into Good Health'.

**What you can do about fructose**

The food industry's main sources of fructose are sucrose from beet or cane, high fructose corn syrup, fruits, and honey. Fructose has the same chemical formula as glucose but its metabolism in the liver into glucose, glycogen, lactate, and fat is the underlying reason why it switches you into fat storage mode. In most countries the main source of fructose is from sucrose, a disaccharide composed of equal portions of fructose and glucose. In the United States another major source of fructose is high-fructose corn syrup (HFCS), which is a commercial liquid product consisting of fructose and glucose in varying proportions, but which in soft drinks is usually 55% fructose and 45% glucose. Foods and drinks that contain fructose in higher or equal amounts to glucose include apple, coconut, grape, honeydew, melon, mango, papaya (paw paw), pear, quince, star fruit, tomato, watermelon, all fruit juices, most sweetened drinks, fruit juice concentrates, dried fruit and tinned fruit. Other items high in fructose are Lebanese cucumber, sweet potato, tomato sauce, tomato paste, chutney, relish, plum sauce, sweet and sour sauce, BBQ sauce, high fructose corn syrup, honey and fortified wines[13].

**Strategy 1** – Eat fruit between meals as a snack and never with other food

**Strategy 2** – Dramatically lower sugar from all sources

If you are seriously overweight then one strategy could be to dramatically lower your sugar intake from all sources. This would result in a low carbohydrate diet and a frequently cited concern is that a low carbohydrate diet has the potential for increased renal disease because of the resulting high protein content of the diet. If the diet is balanced properly with vegetables this is never an issue. A study published in April 2010[14] shows that a very low carbohydrate diet (much lower than the ones we use) does not adversely affect renal function.

**Strategy 3** – Cut out only major sources of fructose and sucrose

For people who are just slightly overweight the strategy could be to just cut out all the major sources of fructose and sucrose in your diet. While food labeling does not always tell you all you need to know about the fructose and sucrose content you can use the internet to check specific foods for their fructose and sucrose content.

**Strategy 4** – Wean yourself off the sweet taste

There is an important thing to remember about the 'sweet' taste. It is addictive and you will need to withdraw from it the same way you would withdraw from any drug. A research paper[15] published in 2007 confirmed what we all know – sugar is incredibly addictive and actually more addictive than cocaine. Overconsumption of sugar-dense foods or beverages is initially motivated by the pleasure of sweet taste, and can be directly compared with drug addiction. The research was carried out on rats but can be related to humans and showed that 94% of animals including even cocaine addicted animals preferred the sweet taste to a dose of cocaine. The research showed that a dependence-like state appeared to be induced by the sugar-dense foods and beverages.

Here are some tips on how to wean yourself off the sweet taste:

- Start with a substitute - Use Herbs & Spices instead of Sugar – when cooking it is often possible to use herbs and spices instead of sugar even if the recipe calls for sugar – when buying processed food look for foods that have used herbs and spices and contain no or little sugar.
- Use cooking techniques that don't take much time but bring out the real flavours of food like stir fries and slow cooking.
- Start appreciating the genuine flavours in whole foods and particularly vegetables – once you start to enjoy eating vegetables your desire for the sweet taste will diminish.
- Shop where 'Whole Foods' are sold – shopping at the butcher, fishmonger and fruit and vegetable barn will provide you with all the healthy ingredients you need for a week of meals and so you don't even need to pass the tempting displays of sweetened food in the supermarket.
- Read labels or check on the internet before you buy any processed food or drink.
- Devote time to enjoying the pleasures of eating the food in front of you and don't allow distractions to spoil this great enjoyment in life.
- Give your palate time to change. You'll gradually lose your taste for excessively sweet foods, so give yourself time to adjust, the end result is fantastic.
- If you live in a country that has traditional healthy foods – then enjoy the experience of following the traditions of your ancestors – don't be fooled by the advertising or packaging of products – this does not make the product healthy. If some of the traditions need a slight modification to make them more healthy then make the change. The recipes for traditional healthy food have been modified steadily over time as knowledge improves. This is not breaking tradition but being part of the tradition of preparing healthy food.

## References

1. Bray GA, et al, 2004, Consumption of high-fructose corn syrup in beverages may play a role in the epidemic of obesity, *American Journal of Clinical Nutrition*, vol. 79, no. 4, pp. 537–543
2. James J, et al, 2004, Preventing childhood obesity by reducing consumption of carbonated drinks: cluster randomised controlled trial, BMJ, 328(7450):1237, doi: 10.1136/bmj.38077.458438.EE
3. James J, et al, 2004, Preventing childhood obesity by reducing consumption of carbonated drinks: cluster randomised controlled trial, BMJ, 328(7450):1237, doi: 10.1136/bmj.38077.458438.EE, PMCID: PMC41660
4. Nseir W, et al, 2010, Soft drinks consumption and nonalcoholic fatty liver disease, World J Gastroenterol, 16(21):2579-88

5.   Stanhope KL, et al, 2009, Consuming fructose-sweetened, not glucose-sweetened, beverages increases visceral adiposity and lipids and decreases insulin sensitivity in overweight/obese humans, *Journal of Clinical Investigation*, 119(5), pp.1322-1334, PMCID: PMC2673878

6.   Kretowicz M, et al, 2011, The Impact of Fructose on Renal Function and Blood Pressure, *International Journal of Nephrology*, Volume 2011, Article ID 315879, 5 pages, doi:10.4061/2011/315879

7.   Z. Ackerman, et al, 2005, Fructose-induced fatty liver disease: hepatic effects of blood pressure and plasma triglyceride reduction, Hypertension, vol. 45, no. 5, pp. 1012–1018,

8.   M. Dirlewanger, et al, 2000, Effects of fructose on hepatic glucose metabolism in humans, *American Journal of Physiology—Endocrinology and Metabolism*, vol. 279, no. 4, pp. E907–E911

9.   Niewoehner CB and Nuttall FQ, 1986, Mechanism of stimulation of liver glycogen synthesis by fructose in alloxan diabetic rats, *Diabetes*, vol. 35, no. 6, pp. 705–711

10.   Youn JH, et al, 1986, Synergism of glucose and fructose in net glycogen synthesis in perfused rat livers, Journal of Biological Chemistry, vol. 261, no. 34, pp. 15960–15969

11.   Tappy L, et al, 2010, Metabolic effects of fructose and the worldwide increase in obesity, *Physiol Rev*, 90(1):23-46

12.   Le K.A, et al, 2009, Fructose overconsumption causes dyslipidemia and ectopic lipid deposition in healthy subjects with and without a family history of type 2 diabetes, *Am J Clin Nutr*, 89(6):1760-5, PMID: 19403641

13.   Shephard SJ, Gibson PR, 2006, Fructose malabsorption and symptoms of irritable bowel syndrome: guidelines for effective dietary management, *J Am Diet Assoc*, 106(10): 1631-1639, PMID: 17000196

14.   Brinkworth GD, et al, 2010 Apr, Renal function following long-term weight loss in individuals with abdominal obesity on a very-low-carbohydrate diet vs. high-carbohydrate diet, *Journal American Diet Association*, 110(4):633-8, PMID: 20338292

15.   Lenoir M, et al, 2007, Intense Sweetness Surpasses Cocaine Reward, *PLoS ONE*, 2(8): e698, doi:10.1371/journal.pone.0000698

# 4   EXERCISE REDUCTION – ITS PART IN THE OBESITY EPIDEMIC

**Summary**

The main point that we want you to take away from this chapter is that regular exercise which is part of your daily routine is essential for good health. Exercise refers to whole of body exercise including muscles, heart, lungs, the gastrointestinal system and the brain. You exercise your gastrointestinal system by giving it whole, unprocessed, foods so that you are chewing and then using peristalsis to move food down the gastrointestinal system and extract what you need from it while cleaning out the system with fibre. Whole of body exercise is a vital part of a healthy lifestyle and should be just automatically done without even needing to think about it. You should always have plenty of energy for physical exercise and after you have exercised you should still have plenty of energy and feel great and be ready for any mental challenge that you want to take.

Of course, if you don't implement the other elements of FEAR reversal then you will not have a high level of energy and you will not be able to make exercise part of your daily routine. So be careful to implement all the aspects of FEAR reversal.

Throughout this chapter we provide you with easy ways to build exercise into your daily routine and have fun doing it.

**Now let's look at what we know about exercise and how we know it**

Let's start by looking at the complete opposite to whole of body exercise - watching television. One interesting study[1] published in August 2011 by researchers at the University of Queensland, Australia showed that on average, every single hour of TV viewed after the age of 25 reduces the viewer's life expectancy by 21.8 minutes. Of course, most people watch TV sitting still and allowing their mind to become absorbed into the television content. Thus while viewing television you are doing the absolute opposite to whole of body exercise. You are not using any muscles and apparently you are not even using much of your brain while you are watching TV. When you combine this level of exercise reduction with the other three elements of FEAR you get a frightening picture of people slowly expanding as they sit and watch television.

Research showing the importance of exercise to good health has been around for a long time and it is pretty obvious that you are not going to burn up much fat if you don't do much exercise. However, by reviewing the research it is possible to focus your exercise in a way that improves your ability to burn fat and works well with the other three aspects of FEAR reversal.

Researchers at the Department of Behavioural Science at the University of Texas School of Public Health conducted a survey[2] showing that 67.6% of respondents did not meet physical activity recommendations of at least 150 minutes per week. The most frequently reported barriers to exercise were 'lack of time', 'very tired', and 'lack of self-discipline'. Removing the other three elements of FEAR will give you the energy for exercise, so the 'very tired' barrier should disappear. Having 'enough time' and 'lack of discipline' are all about gaining control of your life and we have devoted a later chapter on how to go about gaining control of your life.

It would appear that 21 minutes of exercise per day (150 minutes per week) is not very much and really is nowhere near enough to give your body a full work out. When you think about the need for all your muscles, plus lungs and heart to get a good work out you need to allocate at least an hour per day. Even for patients who have experienced heart failure the conventional cardiac rehabilitation program consists of 15 min of warm-up, 30 min of aerobic exercise followed by 15 min calisthenics and researchers have found that by adding pilates to the program the rate of recovery increases even more[3].

Researchers[4] in Greece have shown that exercise is beneficial for all forms of diabetes. Other researchers have demonstrated that exercise improves the quality of life of HIV/AIDS patients[5]. Even patients with advanced stage lung cancer, undergoing chemotherapy were found to have improved outcomes by including exercise training in their treatment protocol[6].

Another study[7] showed that men with depression reduced their symptoms by regular exercise.

So there is little doubt that regular physical exercise improves your health. However, when you look at exercise alone and its effects on weight loss you get conflicting results with some people showing losses, others no effect and others weight gain[8]. The answer is, of course, that FEAR is what made you fat and just reversing one element of FEAR will not get the desired results and you need to have a combined approach and reverse all the elements of FEAR.

## What you can do about exercise

### Strategy 1 – Build exercise into your daily routine

When exercise is part of your daily routine you don't need to think about it and you just exercise automatically. You might find a cheap parking station several blocks away from your work and walk to and from there every work day. Every morning you could take the dog for a walk. You could always use the stairs instead of an elevator. You could walk to the local shops instead of going by car. You could walk to the local newsagent instead of getting your paper delivered. You could set up a cross bar in your garage and do pull ups every morning before breakfast. You could do sit ups before you even get out of bed. You could walk with the kids to school instead of driving them. You could play a sport with the kids as soon as you get home. You could use manual tools instead of electric tools for work around the house (if you look hard enough all the manual tools and appliances are still available, even though you may have to ask your grandparents what they look like). Take up a sport and build the training into your weekly program. Take up dancing and build this into your regular routine. Look for the opportunities and you will find plenty of ways to build exercise into your daily routine.

### Strategy 2 – Replace time watching television with exercise

If you currently watch four hours of television per day, then try cutting this down to two hours per day and use one hour to do physical exercise and the other hour to do mental exercise like playing chess, doing puzzles or playing games with friends and family.

### Strategy 3 – Get professional help

It is recommended that you use the services of a personal trainer or gym instructor or other instructor (pilates, yoga, dance, etc) when developing and learning the exercises as correct body positioning is important in any exercise to ensure you do not develop an injury.

Always start an exercise program at low intensity and slowly increase this on subsequent days, even if you have only stopped exercising for a few days.

As you challenge yourself to walk an extra 20 metres every other day or lift slightly more weights or improve your flexibility, you may feel tightness or stiffness in your muscles that will gradually go away and indicate an improvement in your fitness. However, pain should not be the result of your exercise. If you are experiencing pain then have a professional check your posture and body positioning while exercising to make sure you are not creating an injury - pain is a warning sign of injury and should not be ignored. Find out the best way to do an exercise and practice your technique. Pushing yourself too hard (unless under the supervision of an exercise professional) will invariably lead to injury or burn out and a setback in your progress to improved health.

Do not exercise while you have an acute illness such as a cold or flu as this may worsen the condition.

**Strategy 4 – Interval Training**

As you advance with exercise and build muscle and improve joint functionality as a result of the reversal of all elements of FEAR, it is recommended that you consider interval training (short periods of high exertion followed by slightly longer periods of rest). Research[9] has shown that a well designed interval training schedule can result in your body producing good levels of Human Growth Hormone (hGH) – the hormone that many medical experts regard important for building muscle and possibly is one of the keys to staying young. Interval training when combined with appropriate diet has also been shown to reduce muscle wasting in the elderly[10]. Researchers have also found that low-volume high-intensity interval training can rapidly improve glucose control and induce adaptations in skeletal muscle that are linked to improved metabolic health in patients with type 2 diabetes[11].

**Strategy 5 – Check that your routine covers all aspects of exercise**

As you gradually build exercise into your daily routine check that you are covering all the following areas:

- Aerobic exercise
- Muscle strengthening exercise
- Stretching
- Mental exercise

You may decide to choose a sport that combines a number of these into one activity. Tennis, for example, uses arms and legs, requires you to keep on the move so exercising heart and lungs, exercises your eyes, involves stretching and requires you think about a strategy for winning.

Make sure that you are always strengthening the main muscles in your arms, legs, chest and abdomen as this will generate signals to your body to burn more fat and these exercises will also promote the rebuilding of muscle and bone which will send further signals to your body to burn more fat.

## Strategy 6 – Exercise your gastrointestinal system

Whole foods with fibre like vegetables and whole grains require your gastrointestinal system to work on them to extract what you need and also to work at moving the bulk through your gastrointestinal system. Whole foods including meats require you to chew which is another good work out for your gastrointestinal system as chewing burns energy and sets a number of other processes in motion.

## Strategy 7 – Gain Control of Your Life

If you are having trouble implementing any of the above read through our chapter on how to gain control of your life.

## Strategy 8 – Find the Reason If You Feel Too Tired To Exercise

You should never feel too tired to exercise. If you do, then check that you have undertaken all the aspects of FEAR reversal. If you are still having problems then read through our chapter on 'How to turn disease into good health'.


## References

1.    Veerman JL, et al , 2011, Television viewing time and reduced life expectancy: a life table analysis, *Br J Sports Medicine*, [Epub ahead of print], PMID: 21844603
2.    Bautista L, et al, 2011, Perceived barriers to exercise in Hispanic adults by level of activity, *J Phys Act Health*, 8(7):916-25, PMID: 21885882
3.    Guimaraes GV, et al, 2011, Pilates in Heart Failure Patients: A Randomized Controlled Pilot Trial, *Cardiovasc Ther*, doi: 10.1111/j.1755-5922.2011.00285.x, PMID: 21884019
4.    Kourtoglou GL, 2011, Insulin therapy and exercise, *Diabetes Res Clin Pract*, 93 Suppl 1:S73-7,  PMID: 21864755

5.    Ogalha C, et al, 2011, A randomized, clinical trial to evaluate the impact of regular physical activity on the quality of life, body morphology and metabolic parameters of patients with AIDS in salvador, Brazil, *J Acquir Immune Defic Syndr*, 57 Suppl 3:S179-85,  PMID: 21857315

6.    Quist M, et al, 2011, Safety and feasibility of a combined exercise intervention for inoperable lung cancer patients undergoing chemotherapy: A pilot study, *Lung Cancer*, [Epub ahead of print], PMID: 21816503

7.    Sieverdes JC, et al, 2011, Association between Leisure-Time Physical Activity and Depressive Symptoms in Men, *Med Sci Sports Exerc*, [Epub ahead of print], PMID: 21775904

8.    Cook CM, Schoeller DA, 2011, Physical activity and weight control: conflicting findings, *Curr Opin Clin Nutr Metab Care*, 14(5):419-24, PMID: 21832897

9.    Wahl P, et al, 2010, Effect of high- and low-intensity exercise and metabolic acidosis on levels of GH, IGF-I, IGFBP-3 and cortisol, *Growth Horm IGF Res.*, 20(5): 380-5. PMID: 20801067

10.   Little JP, Phillips SM, 2009, Resistance exercise and nutrition to counteract muscle wasting, *Appl Physiol Nutr Metab*, 34(5):817-28, PMID: 19935843

11.   Little JP, et al, 2011, Low-volume high-intensity interval training reduces hyperglycemia and increases muscle mitochondrial capacity in patients with type 2 diabetes, *J Appl Physiol*, [Epub ahead of print], PMID: 21868679

# 5   ATRIFICIAL TRANS FAT – ITS PART IN THE OBESITY EPIDEMIC

**Summary**

The main point that we want you to take away from this chapter is that artificial trans fats need to be diligently avoided – you can't just trust food labels. Serious diseases have been shown to be started by artificial trans fats when they are as little as 2% of your diet but problems with weight gain can start at lower levels. Artificial trans fats are the worst health disaster that the food industry has ever inflicted on consumers. The consequences of this disaster are still being felt all around the world in waves of aftershocks that we explain in this chapter.

**Now let's look at what we know about Artificial Trans Fats and how we know it**

During the 1960's and 1970's the food industry introduced the artificially created trans fat version of saturated fats into virtually all foods produced by the food industry. The fat tasted the same as the natural cis-saturated fats but was cheap to produce and stored well because their shape allowed them to pack tightly and form solids more easily. From the mid 1970's until the early 2000's virtually all take away food and all packaged food throughout the world contained significant amounts of artificial trans fats.

A research paper[1] published in April 2009 by researchers from the Harvard School of Public Health provides a good summary of the research and how trans fats are a primary cause or contributor to obesity, metabolic syndrome, heart disease and diabetes. The researchers highlight that even with artificial trans fats as low as 2% of the diet you still get a marked increase in disease.

The diseases associated with artificial trans fats are also the starting point for many other serious diseases like cancer. Research pointing out the potential damage caused by artificial trans fats steadily mounted from the early 1980's but was ignored by the food industry and governments until the disaster was so widespread that they couldn't ignore it any longer.

A research study[2] published in 1981 concluded that trans fats were preferentially deposited in adipose tissue and the liver at concentration levels between 2.4% and 12.2% for adipose tissue and between 4% and 14.4% for the liver. The researchers also noted that the trans fats can be incorporated into membrane phospholipids thus altering the packing of the phospholipids. This means that trans fats can alter the physical nature of cells in adipose tissue and the liver as well as the activities of the associated membrane enzymes such as elongase, desaturase and PG syntherase. In simple terms this means that the liver cells that have received trans fats into their outer layer will not function properly as they are no longer able to move substances normally through the tightly packed outer layer. It also means that removing trans fats from fat cells is much more difficult than removing cis fats and consequently weight loss can become very difficult to achieve for some people. The researchers who undertook this study in 1981 didn't recommend the removal of trans fats from foods but gave a very clear indication to food industry scientists and governments that a potential disaster was in its early stages.

After about 20 years of inaction, governments around the world started to take specific actions and most countries now have some controls over artificial trans fats. Unfortunately, some countries like the United States haven't required the removal of trans fats from all foods but require the food to be labeled if the trans fat content is more than 0.5 grams. The label can read zero trans fats if the quantity is less than 0.5 grams which means that you could be unknowingly consuming 0.49 grams of trans fats in four different products and thus consume 1.96 grams of trans fats in a single day. The US Food and Drug Administration recommend that healthy individuals do not exceed a daily maximum of 1.11 grams. There are naturally occurring trans fats in some foods but they occur at such low quantities that they have not been identified as causing any health problems. So it is hard to confirm a safe level for trans fats but for people wanting to lose weight or get healthy then it would seem logical to avoid all artificially created trans fats and just be exposed to the small quantity of naturally occurring ones.

Even with the actions taken to date with artificial trans fats the world is still suffering the following aftershocks caused by the disaster.

## Aftershock 1

We have a whole generation of people incorrectly believing that a low saturated fat diet is essential for good health. When you consider the low amount of artificial trans fats that triggers disease, it immediately throws into doubt all those studies that showed that saturated fats are bad for you. Scientists are trying to recalibrate these studies to see whether saturated fats are still bad for you once you remove the artificial trans fat content. The growing opinion is that naturally occurring saturated fats are not actually bad for you. In a meta-analysis[3], which combined the results of 21 previous studies, researchers found no clear evidence that higher saturated fat intakes led to higher risks of heart disease or stroke. Of course, overconsumption of any food will have detrimental effects on health so this does not mean that you should over consume natural cis saturated fats. Unfortunately, many food companies are continuing to perpetuate the 'low fat' misconception by incorrectly promoting low fat foods as healthy – what they should be promoting is a zero artificial trans fat diet.

Fats actually play an important part in your health and although unsaturated fats are a healthy option they cannot fully replace saturated fats. The important role of fats include:

- Some vitamins (A, D, E and K) are fat-soluble and can only be digested, absorbed and transported in conjunction with fats.
- Fats are also sources of essential fatty acids, an important dietary requirement.
- Fats in your body play a vital role in maintaining healthy skin and hair, insulating body organs against shock, maintaining body temperature, and promoting healthy cell function.
- Fats in your body also serve as energy stores - they are broken down in the body to release glycerol and free fatty acids. The glycerol can be converted to glucose by the liver and thus used as a source of energy. So while we don't want big roles of fat hanging off our bodies we do need some strategic supplies of fat throughout the body.
- Fat also serves as a useful buffer towards a host of diseases. If a substance, reaches unsafe levels in the bloodstream, the body can effectively dilute, or at least maintain equilibrium of, the offending substances by storing it in new fat tissue

When we get to the chapter on 'Reduced Key Nutrients' we will talk about protein. Fats are broken down in the body by enzymes called lipases produced in the pancreas. These enzymes are made from protein and so someone without enough protein to produce enzymes in the pancreas will not be able to properly utilize the fats in their diet. This is another illustration of how all four elements of FEAR must be addressed before you can lose weight and regain good health.

## Aftershock 2

It is a massive effort to remove all artificial trans fats from the world's processed food and takeaway food and many people throughout the world are still consuming dangerous levels of artificial trans fats. If you live in a country that is slow at taking action you need to check for yourself that you are not consuming any artificial trans fats.

## Aftershock 3

Carbohydrates became the substitute for most people decreasing saturated fat in their diets. Now some researchers believe that a high carbohydrate diet is actually worse for your cardiovascular system than a high saturated fat diet[4].

## Aftershock 4

While normal liver cells die and are replaced on a regular basis nobody knows whether a liver cell with artificial trans fats in its outer layer will die and be replaced or whether it will remain as if it were a non-functional type of scar tissue. This raises many unanswered questions such as whether some people have a reduced liver capacity to clear drugs, or turn a pro-drug into an actual functional drug. If you need a drug for an important medical reason then the only way to make sure you are maintaining the desired blood levels is to have regular blood tests. We cannot rely on previous assumptions about drug dose levels because your liver may not be working to full capacity. Reduced liver capacity could be a factor in many diseases as it is hard to think of an aspect of your health that is not influenced by actions of your liver.

## Aftershock 5

Over the last 50 years most countries have been forced to allocate more and more resources to their hospital and medical systems which are failing to cope with the large volume of disease. This has meant that we have a medical system focused on fighting disease (and not winning the battle) instead of being focused on helping people get healthy. Hopefully with the removal of artificial trans fats, and the reversal of the other aspects of FEAR, the pressure can be taken off the world's hospital and medical resources and medical staff can once again have the time to do their job properly and take pride in their valuable skills.

## FOOTNOTE

The properties of any specific fat molecule depend on the particular fatty acids that constitute it. A fat's constituent fatty acids differ in the number of hydrogen atoms that are bonded to the chain of carbon atoms. When a fatty acid has each carbon atom bonded to two hydrogen atoms it is called 'saturated' - meaning they are bonded to as many hydrogen atoms as possible. Saturated fats can stack themselves in a closely packed arrangement, so they can freeze easily and are typically solid at room temperature. When a carbon atom is instead bonded to only one other hydrogen atom and has a double bond to a neighbouring carbon atom – this is called a "monounsaturated" fatty acid. A polyunsaturated fatty acid would be a fatty acid with more than one double bond.

There are two ways the double bond may be arranged: the isomer with both parts of the chain on the same side of the double bond (the cis-isomer), or the isomer with the parts of the chain on opposite sides of the double bond (the trans-isomer, or trans-fat). Most trans fats are commercially produced rather than naturally occurring. The *cis*-isomer introduces a kink into the molecule that prevents the fats from stacking efficiently as in the case of fats with saturated chains. This makes it more difficult for unsaturated cis-fats to freeze - they are typically liquid at room temperature. Trans fats may still stack like saturated fats. Trans fats, however, stack more evenly and this made them popular in production of foods but also created the disease issues.

The primary health risk identified by researchers for trans fat consumption is an elevated risk of coronary heart disease.[3,5,6]

There are two accepted blood tests that measure an individual's risk for coronary heart disease: a) the ratio of LDL cholesterol to HDL cholesterol and the amount of C-reactive protein. LDLs (Low-density lipoproteins) transport cholesterol to the tissues and HDLs (High-density lipoproteins) scavenge excess cholesterol for return to the liver and therefore are protective against arterial disease. Increased levels of LDLs are associated with fatty plaque (atherosclerosis) eventually leading to a more serious cardiovascular disease such as coronary thrombosis of a coronary artery and heart attack, or the same process in an artery to the brain (stroke) or claudication from insufficient blood supply to the legs.

The effect of trans fat consumption has been documented on each as follows:

- Cholesterol ratio: Trans fat behaves like saturated fat by raising the level of LDL, but, unlike saturated fat, it has the additional effect of decreasing levels of HDL. The net increase in LDL/HDL ratio with trans fat is approximately double that due to saturated fat.[7,8] (Higher ratios are worse.)

- C-reactive protein (CRP): A study of over 700 nurses showed that those in the highest quartile of trans fat consumption had blood levels of CRP that were 73% higher than those in the lowest quartile[9]. This meant they were suffering from a high level of internal inflammation which indicates chronic disease.

Consequently it appears that trans fats are a big cause of the increase in heart attack and stroke in developed countries and the food industry must take responsibility as they used artificial trans fats in a wide range of foods. Of course, over consumption of other foods like sugar can also contribute to cardiovascular disease and so the sole blame cannot be placed on trans fats.

Consumption of polyunsaturated fats, on the other hand has been linked by researchers to a decrease in cardiovascular disease.[10]

Thus a well balanced diet that has adequate amounts of both saturated fats and unsaturated fats from natural sources is not likely to provide any risk of cardiovascular disease.

Before we go off the topic of fats and cholesterol we want to debunk another myth about how the cholesterol in eggs is supposedly bad for your health. Research [11,12] has shown that regular egg consumption (2 eggs daily for 6 weeks) has no negative effects on blood cholesterol. The reason is simple – if you live a balanced lifestyle eating natural foods then your body has enough LDLs to carry cholesterol to your cells where it is essential for many body functions including production of hormones and your body has plenty of HDLs to scavenge any surplus cholesterol and bring it back to the liver for processing – none will be left in your arteries to start a process of cardiovascular disease. So once you implement FEAR reversal then egg consumption is not a problem.

## References

1.    Micha R, Mozaffarian D, 2009, Trans fatty acids: effects on metabolic syndrome, heart disease and diabetes, *Nat Rev Endocrinol*, 5(6):335-44, PMID: 19399016

2.    Kinsella JE, et al, 1981, Metabolism of trans fatty acids with emphasis on the effects of trans, trans-octadecadienoate on lipid composition, essential fatty acid, and prostaglandins: an overview, *The American Journal of Clinical Nutrition*, 34: pp2307-2318

3.    Siri-Tarino PW, et al, 2010, Meta-analysis of prospective cohort studies evaluating the association of saturated fat with cardiovascular disease, *Cam J Clin Nutr*, 91(3):535-46, PMID: 20071648

4.    Hu FB, 2010, Are refined carbohydrates worse than saturated fat?, *Am J Clin Nutr*, 91(6): 1541–1542, doi: 10.3945/ajcn.2010.29622, PMCID: PMC2869506

5.    Hu, FB; et al, 1997, Dietary fat intake and the risk of coronary heart disease in women, *New England Journal of Medicine*, 337 (21): 1491–1499, PMID 9366580

6.    Mozaffarian D, et al, 2006, Trans fatty acids and cardiovascular disease, *New England Journal of Medicine*, 354 (15): 1601–13, PMID: 16611951

7.    Ascherio A, et al, 1999, Trans fatty acids and coronary heart disease, *New England Journal of Medicine*, 340 (25): 1994–1998, PMID 10379026.

8.    Gatto L, et al, 2003, Postprandial effects of dietary trans fatty acids on apolipoprotein(a) and cholesteryl ester transfer, *American Journal of Clinical Nutrition*, 77 (5): 1119–1124, PMID 12716661

9.    Lopez-Garcia, E, 2005, Consumption of Trans Fatty Acids Is Related to Plasma Biomarkers of Inflammation and Endothelial Dysfunction, *The Journal of Nutrition*, 135 (3): 562–566, PMID 15735094

10.    Oh K, Hu FB, et al, 2005, Dietary fat intake and risk of coronary heart disease in women: 20 years of follow-up of the nurses' health study, *American Journal of Epidemiology*, 161 (7): 672–679, PMID: 15781956

11.    Katz DL, et al, 2005, Egg consumption and endothelial function: a randomized controlled crossover trial, *International Journal of Cardiology*, 99(1): 65-70, PMID: 15721501

12.    Njike V, et al, 2010, Daily egg consumption in hyperlipidemic adults--effects on endothelial function and cardiovascular risk, *Nutrition Journal*, 9:28, PMID: 20598142

# 6  REDUCED KEY NUTRIENTS – ITS PART IN THE OBESITY EPIDEMIC

**Summary**

The main point that we want you to take away from this chapter is that if you are deficient in any one of a number of key nutrients this is likely to contribute to weight gain and make it extremely difficult to lose weight.  Even though you may consume adequate quantities of a nutrient it is possible that your ability to absorb and transport the nutrient throughout your body has been compromised and consequently this issue also needs to be checked.

The issue of 'reduced key nutrients' is incredibly widespread and this issue is often ignored by people trying to lose weight as well as their health advisors. By the end of this chapter you will be equipped with enough knowledge to check that you are getting all the key nutrients so that you can implement all four aspects of FEAR reversal.

**Not let's look at what we know about key nutrients and how we know it**

## PROTEIN

Protein is the one essential nutrient that you must always check that you are getting in adequate quantities.  Protein gives your body the ingredients needed for every structural and functional aspect of your body.  With protein you build your immune system, your gastrointestinal system, heart muscle, lungs, skeletal muscle and functional things like enzymes, etc, etc.  Eggs, fish, legumes and lean meats are the best sources of protein.  If you are a vegetarian then you will need to make sure that your vegetable and grain combinations are working to give you the full range of protein needed for good health.

Now let's look at why you may be deficient in protein without even knowing it.

Your pancreas makes digestive enzymes from protein and these enzymes are sent down into your small intestine as part of the process of breaking up proteins and helping them to pass through the lining of the gastrointestinal system. Many people get so low in protein that they don't make enough of these digestive enzymes to facilitate the process of digesting and absorbing protein. So even though your diet may be brought back to be adequate in protein you may not be actually receiving these proteins where they are needed. Digestive enzymes are readily available in supplement form from pharmacies and health practitioners so you may need to take some of these with food for a short time to break the cycle.

If you are taking a drug that is a H2 blocker or proton pump inhibitor you are taking a class of drug whose main action is a pronounced and long-lasting reduction of gastric acid production. Gastric acid is produced in cells around the stomach and is needed in the stomach to break down proteins before they leave the stomach so that they will be in a form ready for the action of the digestive enzymes in the small intestine. Research[1] has also shown that the gastric acid barrier not only controls the colonization and growth of oropharyngeal bacteria, but also regulates the population and composition of lower intestinal microflora. Thus lower gastric acid can result in other digestive complications. So if you are taking one of these drugs it is likely that your gastric acid level will be too low to enable you to break down and absorb all the protein that you need and you will be having other gastrointestinal problems. Now H2 blockers or proton pump inhibitors are normally prescribed by medical practitioners to prevent acidic reflux into your oesophagus which is a dangerous condition and can lead to cancer. The primary cause of oesophageal reflux is obesity - i.e. your fat gut putting so much pressure on your stomach that acid is forced back up your oesophagus. So FEAR reversal will mean that you get rid of the fat gut and you can gradually withdraw from the H2 blocker or proton pump inhibitor with your doctor monitoring your progress to make sure you are not at any risk. If you have another cause of oesophageal reflux you may need further assistance to withdraw from this class of drug. During the withdrawal process you may need to use protein powders and other protein sources that need less gastric acid to break them down.

The way your body responds to stress could be another reason why you are not absorbing enough protein from your diet. The fight-or-flight response (short-term stress) goes something like this: When a villager in Africa sees a lion charging at him, for example, the brain sends a signal to the adrenal gland to create hormones called cortisol and adrenaline, which have many different effects on the body, from increasing heart rate and breathing to dilating blood vessels so that blood can flow quickly to the muscles in the legs and slowing digestion. Besides helping our villager run away, this type of acute stress also boosts the immune response for three to five days (presumably to help him heal after the lion takes a swipe at him). Health problems start to arise when you are continuing to respond to stress over an extended period of time as is the case in our modern society with anything from traffic noise to people complaining, having the potential to stimulate the stress response. We know that high cortisol levels have an effect on the digestion process with a possible reduction in the amount of protein absorbed from a meal but this is probably the most under-researched area in nutrition. It is likely that chronic stress creates a stop/start process with some meals working well and the protein gets through while other meals the protein absorbed is small. If you suspect that your stress response is causing a protein absorption problem for you, then the simple answer is to find a supplement containing betaine hydrochloride (i.e. the main ingredient in stomach acid) and also digestive enzymes and take these with your protein meal. There are also medicines that can help modify your stress response or help you adapt to it, so these may be worth investigating as well.

There are many other reasons why you may not be getting enough protein and consistent, thorough investigation is needed to track down things like pancreatic obstruction, lack of carrier proteins for transport of amino acids across the gastrointestinal lining, drinking alcohol with meals, infection with Helicobacter pylori[2] are all risk factors for declining absorption of protein. A variety of drugs can interfere with the process of transporting amino acids through the lining of the gastrointestinal system. Autoimmune destruction of gastric parietal cells is another potential issue. So the answer is FEAR reversal, an end to the obesity epidemic and allowing the medical profession to get back to what they are good at – tracking down the causes of disease.

## VITAMIN D

While protein is the most essential of all the key nutrients, Vitamin D is the key nutrient that most people are likely to have low levels.

Most of what science knows about vitamin D and its importance in your body has been discovered since the year 2003. The widespread campaigns against exposing your skin to sunlight were started long before scientists realised the critical importance of vitamin D to your health. Research varies on the level of vitamin D deficiency but most research suggests that it is high, with 68% to 80% of people being potentially deficient in vitamin D[3,4]. It appears that all cells and tissue in your body have vitamin D receptors[5] and they all need vitamin D for well-being. Vitamin D has been related to the regulation of large numbers of genes in your body and is involved in many of the complex metabolic processes that your body carries out daily including the rate at which you burn fat for energy. One study showed that the greater your body fat the greater was your requirement for vitamin D to remain healthy[6].

Your skin naturally produces your body's supply of vitamin D from direct exposure to bright sun with around fifteen minutes of exposure to 20% of your skin per day regarded as the minimum necessary for good health. Depending on the conditions and the skin type some people may need around an hour of sun exposure so if you are relying on sun exposure as your only source of vitamin D it is best to get some professional advice on how much exposure that you need. Current public health warnings caution against extensive midday sun exposure so it may be better to spend 20 minutes or so earlier in the day. You should have your vitamin D levels checked, particularly after the onset of winter and supplement if needed. When supplementing with vitamin D we recommend that you take it in the form of vitamin D3 because there is some controversy over whether vitamin D2 or any other form of vitamin D can fully substitute for vitamin D3 which is the form produced by your skin. Some scientists believe that the form of vitamin D3 available in supplements is not identical to the form of vitamin D3 that is produced in your skin and that you should not rely on supplements as your only source of vitamin D.

Vitamin D has another key role in that it works in conjunction with protein, vitamin K2 and other nutrients for bone formation and bone remodelling and thus the prevention of osteoporosis. Thus if you are deficient in vitamin D you will not be undertaking much rebuilding of muscle and bone and your body will be receiving signals to store fat instead of using it for these purposes. This is why FEAR reversal requires a thorough check of all your nutrients and the way that your body is utilising them. If, for example, you haven't checked that you are getting adequate amounts of protein then you could be wasting your time supplementing with vitamin D or any other vitamin because your body will not be in a position to utilise the supplement.

## VITAMIN K2

There are three known forms of vitamin K. K1 (Phylioquinone) is sourced from plants, K2 (Menaquinone) is from a bacterial source and K3 (Menadione) is a synthetic form of vitamin K. K3 is usually not recommended as a good source for consumption as its biochemical structure is very different to vitamin K1 and K2 and so is not likely to perform the same functions in your body. Long term use of K3 could actually be harmful and you should only use it under the supervision of a qualified practitioner.

Vitamin K is essential for blood clotting, bone mineralisation and calcium metabolism – three issues frequently found in overweight and obese people [7,8,9]. Currently there are no useful tests for vitamin K levels and consequently clinicians very rarely think about it as an issue.

The best sources of vitamin K1 is broccoli, cabbage, eggs, kale, lettuce, pork, soy beans, spinach or soybean oil and bacterial synthesis in the gut.

It is important to note that K2 is produced by gut bacteria or is available in fermented foods, particularly fermented cheese and the Japanese food natto.

As you undertake FEAR reversal it is likely that you will gradually pick up your vitamin K1 levels, if indeed you were deficient to start with. However, vitamin K2 is another story, as the dietary sources are rarely used in the Western diet. Consequently, people on a Western diet are relying completely on their gut bacteria to produce K2. As we have seen above, it is very common for overweight and obese people to have an imbalance in the gut bacteria levels which reduces the chances that vitamin K2 will be available in adequate quantities.

Researchers[10] from the Molecular Genetics and Naomi Berrie Diabetes Center, at Columbia University College of Physicians and Surgeons, in New York published research which highlights that the amount of fat that you accumulate, and the dietary choices that you are driven to make, can be directed by the microbiota composition of your gastrointestinal system. One of the mechanisms proposed for this is that leptin may mediate regulation of mucus production and, or, inflammatory processes that alter the gut habitat. So an imbalance in your gut bacteria could not only be making you deficient in vitamin K2, it could actually be stimulating you to eat more of what makes you fat.

The body of scientific evidence about vitamin K2 is growing rapidly and some of the key issues in regard to the obesity epidemic are set out below.

The Rotterdam Study[11] highlighted the importance of K2 in a variety of health functions, because it was inversely related to all-cause mortality and showed that people who consume 45 mcg of K2 daily live seven years longer than people getting 12 mcg per day. Data from the Prospect Study[12] with 16,000 people followed for 10 years showed that each additional 10 mcg of K2 in the diet results in 9 percent fewer cardiac events.

Another study[13] demonstrated that vitamin K2 therapy improves bone remodelling in haemodialysis patients with a low intact parathyroid hormone level. A vitamin K2 therapeutic treatment for osteoporosis is approved in Japan. Japanese researchers[14] have been able to demonstrate that fermented soybean (Natto), which is high in K2, is useful for premenopausal women in promoting bone formation. Another group of Japanese researchers[15]have carried out research on rats, showing that vitamin K2 is effective in promoting the healing of severed bones.

It is important to remember that vitamin K2 does not act independently but acts in conjunction with other nutrients. So by reversing all the aspects of FEAR you will start to lose weight and start to put an end to the obesity epidemic and start rebuilding your body. During weight loss we recommend supplementing with vitamin K2 as well as a probiotic so that you improve your gut bacteria but also top up on K2 so that you can kick start a number of processes in your body and burn more fat.

## Co Enzyme Q10

Co Enzyme Q10 (Ubiquinone, Ubidecarenone), or CoQ10 for short, is an antioxidant vitamin used in every cell of the body. Ninety-five percent of the human body's energy is generated by a process which uses CoQ10. Therefore, those organs with the highest energy requirements—such as the heart and the liver—have the highest CoQ10 concentrations. CoQ10 levels can diminish with age, and as a result of dietary inadequacies and various disease states. Also, some drugs, especially a group of cholesterol lowering prescription drugs known as "statins" (Pravachol, Zocor, Lipitor, etc) significantly reduce CoQ10 levels in the body which are, of course, frequently taken by overweight and obese people. While supplementing with CoQ10 is often helpful in weight loss it can interact with some drugs and nutrients, and so it is extremely important that you consult someone qualified in nutritional medicine before taking CoQ10.

## OTHER KEY NUTRIENTS

Our experience with weight loss clients indicates that a number of other key nutrients can be missing in the diet with magnesium and calcium being two examples. Fibre is another key nutrient needed for weight loss as essential compounds are produced during the fermentation of soluble fibre, and insoluble fibre has the ability to increase bulk, soften stool, and shorten transit time through the intestinal tract. Water is another key nutrient needed for weight loss, as having adequate amounts of water is needed for virtually every biochemical action in the body.

All types of chronic disease can block your body from absorbing or transporting key nutrients. So you may need to follow the steps in our chapter on 'Turn Disease into Good Health' to make sure you are not suffering a blockage.

**What you can do about nutrient deficiencies**

**Strategy 1 – Have a professional review your diet**

Someone experienced in nutrition should be able to pick up the key items that are missing from your diet and recommend corrective action.

**Strategy 2 – Supplement for the obvious deficiencies**

As you can see from the above it is highly likely that you will need digestive enzymes, a probiotic, vitamin D3 and vitamin K2 just to kick start the process of rebuilding good health and starting the weight loss process. It is possible that you  may need a few other targeted supplements if your health practitioner identifies other issues.

**Strategy 3 – Drink plenty of water**

The amount of water you need varies between people so you need to do a bit of investigation to see if you are drinking enough.

**Strategy 4 – Include plenty of vegetables in your diet**

Some nutritionists recommend five serves of vegetables per day but we recommend that you go well beyond this and try for six or seven servings per day. The scientific evidence is convincing that vegetables are protective against cancer, coronary heart disease and stroke [16,17]. Vegetables may also play a role in preventing cataracts, diverticulosis, high blood pressure, and types of chronic obstructive pulmonary disease including asthma and bronchitis [16,17].

In addition to reducing your risk of developing disease, vegetables contain good amounts of carbohydrates, vitamins and minerals in combinations that your body needs to give you optimum levels of energy. Vegetables grown locally are likely to be fresh with the best nutrient content – even better if you grow your own. By rotating the variety of vegetables available to us, we can have a varied and balanced diet. When you buy vegetables find out where they have been produced and what farming methods have been used. Organic may be the best choice although you might find that the farmers in your area use very safe practices and have great healthy soils – you will not know unless you investigate. The nutrient value of vegetables can be retained by eating them raw, steaming, stir frying or baking.

Selecting vegetables by colour is a simple way of making sure you get a good variety of nutrients. Try to have at least one serving from every colour every day. One way of dividing vegetables into colours is set out below:

• Green – includes spinach, broccoli, lettuce, asparagus, peas, green beans, cabbage, Brussels sprouts, green olives.
• Orange/yellow – includes carrots, pumpkin, corn, and sweet potato (avoid sweet potato while you are losing weight due to its fructose content).
• White/Brown – includes cauliflower, garlic, ginger, mushrooms, onions, chickpeas, and potatoes (note – it is best to avoid potatoes during weight loss as they contain high levels of starches that may promote fat storage).
• Red – red capsicum, radishes and tomatoes (although you may want to keep the level of tomato consumption down while you are losing weight because it is high in fructose – it is really a fruit and not a vegetable).
• Purple/blue – beetroot, purple asparagus, red cabbage, olives, red onions.
• Multi-coloured – avocado, zucchini, egg plant, and beans can be a variety of colours, celery.
By selecting a good variety of vegetables you are obtaining a good selection of carbohydrates, fats, fibre, protein, water, vitamins, minerals and phytochemicals. The study of phytochemicals in vegetables is progressing rapidly, with scientists uncovering another health improvement aspect, or disease fighting aspect virtually every day.

If you think it is hard to get enough vegetables into your diet here are some simple ideas:

• A stir fry is a simple way of getting a good variety of vegetables in one meal.
• Garlic, ginger, spinach, etc can be added to lots of meals including omelettes and frittatas.
• Increase the variety in salads by adding to the traditional salad vegetables others such as baby spinach, rocket, lightly steamed broccoli, red capsicum, butterbeans or chickpeas.
• Take a salad to work for lunch, instead of buying a takeaway.
• Grate or dice onion, carrot, zucchini, red capsicum and corn into a savoury muffin mixture.
• Have vegetable sticks such as carrot and celery on hand for a healthy snack, and these can be eaten with hummus.

Of course, some vegetables contain fructose and part of the FEAR reversal process is to reduce your fructose consumption as this will put you into fat storage mode. If you are eating whole vegetables you have the advantage that the other ingredients can offset the effects of fructose. You can also research the fructose content of each vegetable in your diet and cut down on the ones with the largest or eliminate them altogether (e.g. tomatoes – which are really a fruit anyway)

## Strategy 5 – Check meal sizes

If you are using animal protein, then a rough guide is that the animal protein should be about the size of the palm of your hand, and represent about one third of the meal. Using the 'palm of your hand' test to represent one third will result in a full meal for most people being the traditional dinner plate size. If you are eating more than a single dinner plate of food then you are probably over eating. For most people the other two thirds of the meal can be vegetables maybe topped with some good fat like olive oil (remember good fat makes you healthy and not fat). The animal protein is likely to contain enough saturated fat for your needs. During weight loss additional carbohydrates like pasta, rice or white potato are likely to exceed your energy needs, and will be stored as fat or reduce your rate of weight loss and so should be avoided. Some people losing weight find they need to increase the protein portion of the meal to be greater than one third. You will need to do a bit of experimenting to find out what works best for you.

## References

1.      Kanno T, et al, 2009, Gastric acid reduction leads to an alteration in lower intestinal microflora, *Biochem Biophys Res Commun*, 17;381(4):666-70, PMID: 19248769

2.      Adamu MA, et al, 2010, Incidence and risk factors for the development of chronic atrophic gastritis: Five year follow-up of a population-based cohort study, *International Journal of Cancer*, PMID: 20503273 [Epub ahead of print]

3.      Pitman MS, et al, 2011, Vitamin D Deficiency in the Urological Population: A Single Center Analysis, *J Urol*, 2011 Aug 17[Epub ahead of print], PMID: 21855943

4.      Gonzalez-Goss M, et al, 2011, Vitamin D status among adolescents in Europe: the Healthy Lifestyle in Europe by Nutrition in Adolescence study, *Br J Nutr*, Aug 17:1-10. [Epub ahead of print], PMID: 21846429

5.      Makariou S, et al, 2011, Novel roles of vitamin D in disease: what is new in 2011?, *Eur J Intern Med*, ; 22(4):355-62, PMID: 21767752

6.      Arunabh S, et al, 2003, Body fat content and 25-hydroxyvitamin D levels in healthy women, *J Clin Endocrinol Metab*, 88(1):157-61, PMID: 12519845

7.      Koshiharay Y, et al, 2003, Vitamin K stimulates osteoblastogenesis and inhibits osteoclastogenesis in human bone marrow cell culture, *Journal of Endocrinology*, 176(3):339-48, PMID 12630919

8.      Ishida Y, 2008, Vitamin K2, *Clinical Calcium*, 18(10):1476-82, PMID 18830045

9.      Yamauchi M, et al, 2010, Relationships between undercarboxylated osteocalcin and vitamin K intakes, bone turnover, and bone mineral density in healthy women, *Clinical Nutrition*, PMID: 20332058

10.     Ravussin Y, et al, 2011, Responses of Gut Microbiota to Diet Composition and Weight Loss in Lean and Obese Mice, *Obesity* (Silver Spring), 2011 May 19. [Epub ahead of print], PMID: 21593810

11.     Geleijnse J, et al, 2004, Dietary Intake of Menaquinone is Associated with a Reduced Risk of Coronary Heart Disease: The Rotterdam Study, *The American Journal of Nutritional Sciences*, 134:310-3105

12.     Gast GC, et al, 2009, A high menaquinone intake reduce the incidence of coronary heart disease, *Nutr Metab Cardiovasc Dis*, 19(7):504-10, PMID: 19179058

13.     Ochiai M, et al, August 2010, Vitamin K(2) Alters Bone Metabolism Markers in Hemodialysis Patients with a Low Serum Parathyroid Hormone Level, *Nephron Clin Pract*, 117(1):c15-c19, PMID: 20689320

14.     Katsuyama H, et al, 2004, Promotion of bone formation by fermented soybean (Natto) intake in premenopausal women, *J Nutr Sci Vitaminol* (Tokyo), 50(2):114-20

15.     Iwamoto J, et al, March 2010, Vitamin K2 promotes bone healing in a rat femoral osteotomy model with or without glucocorticoid treatment, *Calcit Tissue Int*, 86(3):234-41, PMID: 20111958

16.     Van Duyn MA, Pivonka E, Overview of the health benefits of fruit and vegetable consumption for the dietetics profession: selected literature, *J Am Diet Assoc*, 2000, 100 (12): 1511-21, PMID: 11138444

He K, et al, 2004, Changes in intake of fruits and vegetables in relation to risk of obesity and weight gain among middle-aged women, *Int J Obes Relat Metab Disord*, 28 (12): 1569-74, PMID: 15467774

# 7  GAINING CONTROL OF YOUR LIFE

**Summary**

The key point that we want you to take away from this chapter is that there are things that you can do that will help you gain control of your life.  If you think that it is just too hard for you to implement the steps to overcome FEAR, then this chapter is for you.  Another issue to remember is that nobody else will reverse the aspects of FEAR for you; it is something that you have to decide to do yourself.  You just have to look at how long it took for food scientists and governments to take any action in regard to artificial trans fats to know that nobody else is going to reverse FEAR for you.

**Now let's look at some of the ways to gain control of your life**

First we need to look at something that works against us making changes and often prevents us from taking action to implement the changes needed.  This process is actually one of the most important mechanisms we have in our body and it is called "Homeostasis"

Homeostasis is the condition of equilibrium or balance in the body's internal environment, due to the ceaseless interplay of the body's many regulatory processes.  Every structure in the body, from the cellular level to overall body systems, contribute in some way to keeping the internal environment of the body within normal limits.  As an example of one of the many things monitored is blood glucose levels, which is maintained between 70 and 110 milligrams of glucose per 100 millilitres of blood.

To protect the internal environment, the body will detect undesirable substances entering the skin, nose or gastrointestinal system and mount a defence. Most often the nervous system and the endocrine system, working together or independently, provide the needed corrective measures. Our modern chemical filled environment makes constant demands on these systems and the mechanisms of homeostasis just never stops working in your body. This means you are constantly in a state of feeling OK, even if you are grossly overweight of suffering a chronic disease.

Our own body mechanisms can create a misconception of good health. As you put on a few extra kilograms, then our body makes the corrective actions to make our heart pump faster, etc to keep things in balance. The skin and fat tissues are often used as temporary storage places for dangerous chemicals, until our liver or kidneys can assemble the required enzymes, or other proteins to deal with the offending substance. So in overweight people with low protein levels or other nutrient deficiencies these stored toxins become "time bombs" just waiting to go off. If you were to only reverse some of the elements of FEAR and started to lose some weight your body would pick up that toxins were being released into the blood from fat cells that couldn't be dealt with properly by a liver low in key nutrients, or some other issue. Having detected the dangerous release of toxins, your body would use the tools of homeostasis to put you back into fat storage mode to protect you from harm.

So the first issue to recognise in gaining control of your life is that you have to be smart about the weight loss process. By implementing all the elements of FEAR reversal you will be steadily losing weight and your body will use the mechanisms of homeostasis to gradually accept the thinner you as the new normal – the new feeling of OK. The good thing about implementing all the elements of FEAR reversal at the same time is that you put yourself into fat burning mode and immediately create a feeling of plenty of energy. This was one of the most surprising and exciting discoveries that we made when we first started applying the FEAR reversal process to ourselves and our clients. This feeling of plenty of energy becomes your new normal and you start to use homeostasis for your gradual weight loss and gradual health improvement.

Now let's look at some specific actions that you can take to gain control of your life.

### Strategy 1 – Analyse your own behaviour

By analysing your own behaviour you may discover that you have built in 'Coping Mechanisms' that are actually designed to stop you changing. Sometimes it is also necessary to look at the coping mechanisms that others around you are using, as much of your behaviour may be in response to those around you. Coping mechanisms are patterns of behaviour that we develop which help us deal with the world around us and allow us the feeling of comfort and normality (i.e. a mental form of homeostasis). When you visit your neighbourhood supermarket you tend to deal with the situation in a fixed pattern – you go down the same isles and pick up from the same shelves the same products that you buy every week. So you have developed a coping mechanism for dealing with the supermarket. To implement FEAR reversal you will definitely have to address this coping mechanism and work out a new way of coping with the weekly shopping. Other negative patterns of behaviour can develop that worsen our health condition, while positive coping mechanisms will enable us to easily manage the changes needed to steadily improve our health.

Some examples of negative coping mechanisms are:

- Drama patterns – 'the car has just been repossessed', 'the dog died', 'someone cut me off on the road'. Whenever life threatens to go smoothly a little voice inside says "this can't be right" and to prove it another drama quickly arises.
- Sickness patterns – as soon as good health is achieved another illness arises to prove that 'you are always sick'.
- Indispensable patterns – 'as soon as you train someone they leave', 'you are the only one that can do a job properly', 'people are lazy, they never do their job properly'. These all arise to prove that you are 'indispensable' when, in fact, the world will keep going quite happily whether you are around or not. To reinforce this negative pattern of behaviour people will often invent false standards of what is a good job just to prove that they are the only person who can do the job.
- Mess patterns – constantly living in a mess so that you can never find what you want or, alternatively, you are the only person who can find what you want. This is a way of coping with the reality but always leads to failure.
- Cleanliness patterns - constantly cleaning can be a coping mechanism that blocks out other thoughts just as constantly being messy has the same result. A person who constantly cleans never achieves much else than a temporarily clean environment. Living in a clean environment is actually good and healthy but obsessing about it to the point where you don't have enough time to implement key elements of FEAR reversal creates a problem. So gaining control of your life may often require us to learn new patterns of behaviour that become our new coping mechanisms. Whenever we decide to change, we will always be challenged and meet resistance. Remember that the old pattern of behaviour has taken a long time to build up and is now effectively managed by your subconscious - change will not be easy. The week you decide to adopt a healthy FEAR reversal program you can bet you

will receive a number of invitations to dinners, cocktail parties, birthday parties, etc, just to see if you are serious about making the change.

So to make sure that the change is effective you may need to use some more of the other techniques and strategies we have listed below.

## Strategy 2 – Develop a plan

Having a simple plan of what you want to achieve in your life gives you incredible drive. The feeling of having a purpose in life gives you a positive mind set which helps offset any negatives that may be around you. The nightly news that we see or hear is often so full of negatives that you could easily believe that the world is a terrible place full of bad people. Once you develop a plan for yourself it becomes a lot easier to put things in perspective and see that the negative news items are actually only about a very small portion of the world's population. If you get the opportunity to travel around the world you will start to realise that most people and places are not actually that bad and most people are actually working together to make the world a better place. When you develop a plan for your life and set some objectives, you will quickly see that you can fit into this positive world of people working together to build a better world.

## Strategy 3 – Implement Time Management Techniques

Common reasons given for not implementing a weight loss program are 'very tired', 'not enough time', and 'lack of self-discipline'. Reversing all the elements of FEAR puts you into fat burning mode and creates lots of energy so the 'very tired' reason disappears. Time management techniques can be used to address 'not enough time' and 'lack of self-discipline'. So here are some actions that you may find useful:

- Focus – the most important reality of life is that 'What you focus on is what you get'. So if you focus on FEAR reversal you will achieve weight loss, lots of energy and become healthy – you have to decide that this is your major focus.
- Use a 'To Do List'. Pick the hardest job on the list or the one you dislike doing and do it first. Getting this job out of the way will reduce stress for the rest of the day and make doing the other things feel easy. If you find exercise the hardest thing to implement you might decide to do this first thing every morning, so that you feel good for the rest of the day that you are making progress.
- Break a major job down into simple tasks. Doing each small simple task is a lot less stressful and easier to manage than working on one major job and never getting it finished. You will now see yourself steadily moving towards

your objective one step at a time – so if you are allocated a major job at work which is very important to your career and you definitely want to do it and this may reduce your time available for FEAR reversal, then you need to break the new major job down into smaller parts and address the key issues first so that you can demonstrate you are making progress. This will give you plenty of time to fit in the FEAR reversal tasks into your daily routine.

• Train and delegate. Many people think that they have to do every chore in the house or every key job in the work environment simply because they have experienced a situation in the past where someone has failed to do something properly. If you think like this you will never have time for FEAR reversal. You need to develop skills in training and delegating so that you will have time for the most important task in your life – getting healthy with FEAR reversal. When you train a person to do part of your work, make sure that you are confident that they really understand what to do and the outcomes expected, then leave them to it. You may need to occasionally check their output and do some retraining but your life will become a lot less stressful the more you do this. This works equally at home as well as at work - train the kids to make their beds and clean their rooms - check on them occasionally and praise their good work and retrain them if the results are not good.

• Keep life simple - always eliminate unnecessary complications - the simple ways of doing something are always the most effective and create the least stress and make more time available for implementing FEAR reversal.

• Take notes when important matters come up - you can then deal with these issues when you have time and your mind can be free for the more immediate issues. Notes keep your mind free to focus on the most important issue in front of you – your health and FEAR reversal

• Always be prepared - planning and preparation can always increase the amount of time we have available for the important things in life. Plan the key things you need to do at home and at work - focus on these and not all the minor issues that may arise to distract you.

• Take time to choose your response - if you are faced with an irate person you can choose whether you want to remain calm or you want to blow off steam like them. Either response may be appropriate. The important issue is that you have made the choice in advance and afterwards you don't need to dwell on the issue. You can quickly move on and focus back on the key issue – FEAR reversal. Remember one of the most important realities of life – 'What you focus on is what you get'. Focus on FEAR reversal and you will achieve your goal.

• Build your self-worth. As you implement FEAR reversal you will start to look healthier and may even receive a few positive comments. Simply say 'Thank You' to positive complements as this builds your self-worth without sounding like you were just elected as President. Another technique is to praise in public and criticise in private. Praising a person in public for something that has been well done will add to their self-worth as well as your self-worth. Telling someone about a poor outcome in private will give you the opportunity to talk confidentially about the issues and will keep both of you positive about the outcomes and thus diminishing the level of stress or embarrassment involved. This applies equally at home as well as at work – tell children about poor outcomes in private – not in front of other children or their friends.

• Learn to say "No". Over-commitment will almost always create more stress for you and everyone around you and leave little time for important issues like FEAR reversal. Know your limitations and work within them. By saying "No" to others when something cannot realistically be achieved is being honest and creating certainty. You can then work with the person wanting to delegate work to you to find another way of achieving the outcome without you losing the time needed for your important goals.

• Be alert to procrastination in yourself and in others. Look for the reason that you or someone else is procrastinating and find a way of overcoming the issue.

• Don't be overwhelmed by emails, face book activities or paperwork - sort out what is important and get rid of the rest. Look at ways of minimising what comes to you on a daily basis. Remember – 'What you focus on is what you get'. You now have the tools to focus on losing weight and being healthy so make this your major focus.

## Strategy 4 - Learn to Listen

Listening to another person very carefully so that you really understand what they are talking about is the best compliment that you can give to another person and will make your life incredibly easy and stress free. If you really understand the people around you then you will not be stressed by their behaviour or do things unintentionally that create negative situations. You can also explain your situation in terms that the other person will appreciate. So by listening you become an effective communicator. Effective communication is one of the keys to success in life and will help you implement FEAR reversal. This is particularly important when you live with a group of people and you are the first one of the group to learn about FEAR reversal and want to implement it. The others may not be enthusiastic about the change and may actually sabotage your efforts. So it is very important to fully understand the people around you so that you can implement FEAR reversal in ways that creates the least difficulties for them. When others see the positive results in you they will then be enthusiastic to make the changes as well, provided you communicate in a way that they can relate to and feel positive about.

## Strategy 5 - Think Win/Win

Life doesn't have to be full of situations where one person gets what they want at the expense of another person. By always thinking 'win/win' you will be looking for ways that you can achieve what you want to and allow other people also to achieve what they want to at the same time. This may require a bit of thought but once you get into the habit of thinking like this, it is amazing how quickly effective solutions arise. When you combine the 'win/win' thought pattern with the effective communication you get by 'Learning to Listen' you may find that many people around you also want to participate in FEAR reversal. You may find that all the people around you become an effective support group as you and they go through the process of getting healthy with FEAR reversal.

## Strategy 6– Stress Reduction

We have discussed stress in many ways throughout this book and FEAR reversal plus some of the techniques mentioned above will contribute to making your life less stressful. The following are a few other ideas that may also help reduce stress:

- Have more fun – doing things that you enjoy will help you to relax.
- Express your feelings – unexpressed emotions are the building blocks of stress, pain, and illness.
- Get good sleep – poor sleep or sleep habits do not let your body really rest, discharge tensions and recharge.
- Learn relaxation exercises – these can help reduce stress through letting go of mental stresses and experiencing moments of inner peace.
- Develop good relationships – those who love and accept you, and will advise but not judge you, are your true friends.

## Strategy 7 - Visualisations & Affirmations

We have talked about making FEAR reversal the key objective in your life. Sometimes you have to convince your subconscious that you really do want to achieve this goal. We have developed the following technique that you can use to convince your subconscious that FEAR reversal is your new goal. After achieving the great health and energy that goes with FEAR reversal you may want to use this technique to achieve other things in your life.

Visualisation is a matter of picturing something in your mind. Affirmations are basically words that you repeat to yourself that focus your attention on a particular topic or outcome (they must be clear and precise to be effective). Meditation is a technique of stilling the mind.

For our clients we have combined visualisation, affirmation and meditation into one powerful technique. We call it – 'Perpetual Mind Rejuvenation'. In addition to our weight loss clients we also use this technique for our clients following our anti-aging program called "Perpetual Rejuvenation" (visit us at www.natmed4u.com for more information about our healthy anti-aging program).

The following is an example of how 'Perpetual Mind Rejuvenation' works. As you become experienced in the technique you can use it to achieve many positive outcomes in your life.

Find a quiet spot, sit still and use your mind as follows:

First count the number one to yourself slowly until all thoughts have gone and you are focusing only on the number one.

Next imagine red energy is coming from the earth below your feet and rising up into your legs and that this energy is giving you the stamina you need for today.

Feel the red energy convert to orange energy and allow it to rise up through your body and balance all the hormones in your body so you feel stable and energetic.

Now allow yellow energy from the sun to enter your body through your abdomen and feel it nourish your digestive system including your liver and pancreas.

Next breathe in the green energy of the trees and allow the oxygen to travel to every part of your body.

Imagine the gentle pounding of the ocean and add this blue energy to the blue energy of the sky and allow this blue energy to enter through your throat and let it travel down your spine relaxing each nerve in your body. When the blue energy reaches your toes allow it to travel back up your spine to your face and allow your face to relax and glow with vitality.

Next allow purple energy from the universe to enter through the top of your head so that you now feel totally connected with the whole universe and the knowledge of the universe is freely available to you.

Now allow your whole body to glow with a violet energy that allows you to fully connect with every aspect of the universe.

Finally, while you are fully connected to the universe allow whatever it is you desire to flow into your body – such as weight loss, perfect health, the cure of a disease, meeting the right person, wealth, happiness, development of a specific aspect of your business, removal of a bad habit, adoption of a good habit, etc, etc – but remember that you are using a powerful tool so select what you want carefully and only focus on one thing at a time (one thing in one session).

You can select the words for this final step in the form of an affirmation such as 'My healing has already begun', 'I have more energy every day', 'My muscles are growing stronger as my fat reduces', 'I am willing to change', 'I love life', 'I love my body'.

Before you begin a Perpetual Mind Rejuvenation exercise think carefully about what it is that you most need to change in your life or what is most needed to add to your life to improve it. The objective can be simple or complex and the benefit does not necessarily have to be for you – your objective could be to improve your skill at helping others. When you establish your objective then carefully develop a phrase that explains it. This phrase should be absolutely clear to anybody who hears it so that it is absolutely clear what you want to happen.

You may want to identify the aspect of your behaviour that they want to change and then define a new clear way of coping and use this as your affirmation. An example of an affirmation to change is "I will replace my drama coping mechanism with a 'to do' list which is always up to date with priorities allocated and I am successfully completing the next most important job – life is never a drama for me"

Money is an incredibly important issue for most people in the Western world. So let's have a look at how you would use the technique to improve your financial situation. A phrase like 'I want more money' is not clear as this could mean one cent more, one dollar more, etc. However, a phrase like "My income will increase to $150,000 per annum by June next year" is absolutely clear. Be careful, though, that this is an achievable goal and that you have the health, energy and skills to achieve it. If your starting point is no job at all then you will need to start with an objective of getting a job. If you need more energy you might start with 'My energy levels will improve so that I can work 8 hours a day without getting tired or slowing down' or 'My skill levels will improve so that I am worth $100,000 a year in income' and then, at a later stage, when you have achieved the $100,000 a year level move up to $150,000.

Remember the whole Perpetual Mind Rejuvenation exercise should only focus on one thing at a time and it should be absolutely clear what you are trying to achieve. You are training your subconscious to fully believe your new focus. Also remember that good health is the basis for achieving all other objectives and your initial focus with Perpetual Mind Rejuvenation exercises should be on FEAR reversal and health improvement.

# 8 TURN DISEASE INTO GOOD HEALTH

**Summary**

The key point that we want you to take away from this chapter is that many people who have been exposed to FEAR for a long period of time are now in a state of serious disease. In addition to removing FEAR from their lives, these people may also need the assistance of targeted medications prescribed by medical practitioners. If you are in this position then you can follow the steps we outline in this chapter to get in control of your disease by using the best resources available. FEAR reversal may just buy you the time you need to regain good health and be completely free of disease.

**Now let's look at this issue in more detail**

The following are the steps to turn a disease state into good health

**Step 1 – Reverse all the elements of FEAR**

No matter what your condition, even if you have untreatable terminal cancer FEAR reversal will have health benefits. Your condition might be so severe that you have gone all the way from being overweight to now being underweight and wasting away. The reversal of FEAR may actually improve your health enough so that your doctors can reconsider their treatment options. After your health improves, you may find that your body is functioning well enough that the doctors can now give you a course of chemotherapy or the cancer may have reduced enough for it to become operable.

## Step 2 – Monitor your symptoms

An important issue with chronic disease is to monitor all aspects of your health as you implement the FEAR reversal process. The following is a checklist that we use to monitor the progress of our clients. We have this checklist available on-line so that you can monitor your progress with a graph showing how you are changing on major symptoms over time (at www.perpetualrejuvenation.com) – there is a small fee involved and you also gain access to up to date information about health improvement.

We score each symptom from 1 to 10 with the following meaning:

- 10 = Never or almost never have the symptom
- 8 = Occasionally have it, effect is not severe
- 6 = Occasionally have it, effect is severe
- 3 = Frequently have it, effect is not severe
- 1 – Frequently have it, effect is severe
- The numbers between give you a bit of flexibility if you feel your symptom fits between the definitions with the lower the number the more the frequency or severity of the symptom.

### Digestive Tract Symptoms

- Indigestion or abdominal discomfort/ pain
- Heartburn – episodic or recurrent
- Nausea or vomiting
- Diarrhoea – episodic or recurrent
- Constipation – episodic or recurrent
- Abdominal bloating – episodic or recurrent
- Flatulence – burping or passing gas

### Appetite/ Eating behaviour

- Loss of appetite
- Food cravings
- Binge eating/ drinking or compulsive eating
- Rapid weight gain

### Head

- Faintness or light headedness
- Headaches

- Dizziness or vertigo
- Insomnia or sleep disturbance

## Ears

- Ears are itchy
- Earache or ear infection
- Ringing or buzzing in ears
- Hearing loss or blocked ears

## Eyes

- Bags or dark circles under eyes
- Watery or itchy eyes
- Swollen, reddened or sticky eyelids
- Blurred or tunnel vision or visual disturbances (does not include near of fat-sightedness)

## Nose

- Dripping from nose or excessive mucus production
- Stuffy nose or nasal discharge
- Sinus congestion or sinus infection
- Hay fever or sneezing attacks

## Mouth/Throat

- Sore throat, hoarseness, loss of voice
- Chronic coughing or clearing of throat
- Frequent gagging or difficulty swallowing
- Swollen or discoloured tongue, gums, lips
- Mouth ulcers or sore gums
- Grinding teeth at night

## Lungs

- Chest congestion or productive chest cough
- Shortness of breath or difficulty breathing
- Recurrent or chronic bronchitis
- Asthma – wheezing or coughing spasms

## Heart

- Irregular of skipped heartbeat
- Rapid or pounding heartbeat
- Chest pain

## Skin

- Acne
- Hives, rashes or allergy reaction
- Dry skin
- Hair loss
- Flushing or hot flushes
- Excessive sweating
- Psoriasis

## Joints/muscles

- Feeling or weakness or tiredness
- Pain or aches in muscles
- Pain or aches in the joints or arthritis
- Stiffness or limitation of movement

## Energy/Activity

- Fatigue, sluggishness or lethargy
- Apathy or loss of motivation
- Hyperactivity or restlessness

## Mind/ Cognition

- Learning difficulties
- Poor memory
- Confusion, poor comprehension
- Poor concentration
- Poor physical coordination
- Difficulty in making decisions
- Stuttering or stammering or slurred speech

## Emotions/Feelings

- Mood swings
- Anxiety, fear or nervousness
- Anger, irritability or aggressiveness
- Depression

## General Signs & Symptoms

- Reproductive/hormonal issues
- Recent illness or recurrent illness
- Underweight or rapid weight loss
- Fluid or water retention
- Frequent or urgent urination
- Genital itch or discharge

As you implement the FEAR reversal process you can complete the checklist weekly or every second week and then check how you are progressing. After about 2 months of implementing FEAR reversal you should have a pretty good idea from the checklist which symptoms are improving and which symptoms seem to be blocking your progress. Continue monitoring as you complete the other steps.

## Step 3 – Review the drugs and other medicines you are taking

With the billions of dollars that have been spent on drug development there is at least one drug for virtually every aspect of every chronic condition, which means that most people with a chronic illness will end up taking a cocktail of drugs. When doctors prescribe drugs for an aspect of a chronic condition they rarely tell you about the side effects of long term use of the drug. Long term use here means that you are taking a drug continually for more than 3 months. The reason they usually don't tell you about the side effects is that people start to anticipate or expect the side effect, so sometimes no knowledge is better. However, the reality is that many of the symptoms that you are experiencing on your list of symptoms are likely to be side effects of the drugs you have been taking long term. To find this out just go onto the internet and Google the drug side effects. The most reliable websites for side effects are either run by doctors or the drug company themselves. So if FEAR reversal is not eliminating all your symptoms and the symptom is one of the ones listed as a drug side effect for a drug you are taking, you can discuss this drug with your doctor to see if you can ease off it as your health continues to improve.

After you compile your drug list you should add in the supplements, over the counter medicines and any natural remedies that you are also taking. You can then use the internet to look for interactions between the drugs themselves, between the drugs and other medicines and supplements, and also interactions between the supplements and alternative medicines you are taking. When we assist clients with this review we invariably find that some of the symptoms they are experiencing are actually caused by interactions between what they are taking. With the interaction knowledge you may be able to eliminate many more of your symptoms.

## Step 4 – Encourage your body to heal itself

Steps 1, 2 and 3 above are all targeted at encouraging your body to heal itself. Another action you can now take is utilising the steps we outlined in our chapter on 'Gaining Control of Your Life'. All the actions listed in that chapter will help mentally and physically indicate to your body that you want it to heal.

Express your emotions – it is OK to be 'pissed off' that you have cancer or any chronic disease – be positive when you feel positive.

See if one of the mind body medicine techniques helps you – if not, don't persist. So check out psychotherapy, support groups, meditation, imagery, hypnosis, biofeedback, yoga, dance therapy, music and art therapies, prayer and mental healing. None of these will work as a sole treatment protocol but they can be a great support to other treatments.

## Step 5 – Avoid fad cures and stay under the supervision of qualified medical practitioners

Fad 'cures' sold on the internet or provided by non medical practitioners are highly unlikely to work and may actually make your condition worse. So let your doctors work on the cures while you work on getting healthy.

## Step 6 – Tone down your objectives

If the medical profession says that your malignant tumour cannot be removed or completely eradicated, accept this as the new reality and make your objective to be healthy and allow your body to manage the tumour so that you are effectively 'living with cancer', or living with whatever chronic disease that you have. The concept of trying to kill every cancer with external assistance, or eliminate every chronic disease, may actually be counterproductive and it may be better to get your body healthy enough so that your body can manage the situation. By doing it this way you buy yourself time by living within the limitations the illness has placed on you.

## Step 7 – Research your disease and monitor developments

If steps 1 to 6 have improved your health and bought you time, then you now have the time to look at your disease in a lot more detail. You don't need to have a degree in medicine to research and understand your disease. You will find the internet an invaluable resource in explaining how your disease works, the alternative treatments and what research is going on in this area. You are now in control of your disease instead of it being in control of you. You are now in a position to decide what is best for you and you can discuss alternatives with your medical practitioner. If you find that your medical practitioner doesn't have the time to discuss alternatives with you then it may be time to shop around for a medical practitioner who does have the time and the expertise.

## Step 8 – Eliminate some common problems that may have been overlooked in the above process

With the time and knowledge that you have gained in steps 1 to 7, it may be worth looking at some of the following issues.

## TOXINS & DETOXIFICATION

There is a growing body of research indicating that the amount of toxins that our body has to deal with is increasing steadily. One study[1] in the United States ranked polycyclic aromatic hydrocarbon, benzene, acetaldehyde, and 1,3-butadiene as posing the greatest risk for cancer coming from outdoor air sources, whereas indoor air sources of cancer risk were primarily from chloroform, formaldehyde, and naphthalene risks.

The key to good health in this polluted environment is to have our body systems capable of dealing with the toxins, and disposing of them effectively. One of the organs that is key in this process is the liver. Liver detoxification of toxins happens in two phases. Phase 1 comprises mainly the cytochrome P450 super family of enzymes that binds with the foreign compound. Phase 2 involves the conversion of these compounds into water soluble compounds that can be excreted through the urine or bile. If the toxin arrives in the gastrointestinal system, healthy intestinal cells are also able to trigger phase 1 detoxification. Having a healthy gut flora is also essential to maintaining and supporting the detoxification process.

At the Perpetual Wellbeing Clinic we support the detoxification process by using nutrients that support the rejuvenation of the gastrointestinal cells, the liver cells and also support maintenance of a balanced gut flora. In our modern polluted environment this support process needs to be ongoing, and so it has been included in our one week per month healthy anti-aging program, thus helping our clients maintain their good health for the long term.

Research[2] published in January 2010 links Perfluorooctanoic acid (PFOA) and perfluoroctane sulphonate (PFOS) with people who have current thyroid disease.  PFOA and PFOS are compounds with many industrial and consumer uses including most non-stick cookware and stain and water resistant coatings for carpets and fabrics.  So if you already have thyroid disease then it is important that you avoid items containing PFOA and PFOS.

For the rest of us, this is another reason why we need to maintain our health in pristine condition.  With our gastrointestinal system, liver and kidneys in top working order we have a good chance of detoxifying and removing from our bodies all the environmental toxins as they arrive.

## Some ideas for reducing your exposure to toxins

The toxic load on your body can be reduced but not eliminated by implementing some of the following ideas:

- Reduce the amount of scented products you have in your home or office – including perfumes, colognes, after-shaves, personal-care products, air fresheners, etc.  Be careful about certain 'unscented' products that use 'masking fragrance' to cover up the original fragrance, as these are very toxic.
- See if you can find unscented and environmentally friendly washing powders, fabric softeners, bleaches, detergents, etc.
- Be careful about the use of pesticides, fungicides, herbicides, and fertilizers. Pesticides can contain neuro-toxins (affect the central nervous system) – not something you want to spray on yourself or be breathing in while you are asleep.
- See if you can find non-toxic cleaning products and personal-care products.
- Consider installing water filters - either the reverse osmosis type or a water distillation system may be most effective.
- Eat organic food (food grown without pesticides or fertilizers) as often as possible.
- Wash all vegetable and fruits unless you are going to peel them, even organic produce.
- Avoiding processed foods will considerably cut down your toxic load.
- Check the clothing and other fabrics that you buy or have in your house to make sure they have not been treated with a toxic substance.  Some

'permanent press' or 'wrinkle resistant' fabrics have been treated with formaldehyde. You want to keep your exposure to this toxic substance to an absolute minimum. Formaldehyde is likely to be in resins and other materials in your house or office[1] so don't add more exposure.

• Store food in glass containers as much as possible and avoid food and water stored in plastics, plastic wrap, polystyrene and other substances containing styrene. One study[3] found that styrene continuously leached from plastic water bottles making them less safe than unfiltered drinking water.

• Open your windows as often as possible. Even in the most polluted cities, the outdoor air has been found to be less toxic than the indoor air.

## References in Regard to Toxins

1.    Loh MM, et al, 2007, Ranking cancer risks of organic hazardous air pollutants in the United States, *Environ Health Perspect*, 115(8):1160-8, PMID: 17687442

2.    Melzer D, et al, 2010, Association Between Serum Perfluoroctanoic Acid (PFOA) and Thyroid Disease in the NHANES Study, *Environ Health Perspect*, [Epub ahead of print], PMID: 20089479

3.    Ahmad M, Bajahlan AS, 2007, Leaching of styrene and other aromatic compounds in drinking water from PS bottles, *J Environ Sci (China)*, 19(4): 421-6, PMID: 17915704

## ALLLERGIES

An allergy is a hyperactive response of the immune system to certain substances that are 'foreign' to our bodies. These substances are called allergens, and they can range from food and pollen to drugs and dust and can quite frequently occur in combination. Allergies are something we seem to acquire throughout life, and some people are more susceptible than others. The entry point to our bodies for allergens is usually the upper respiratory tract or the gastrointestinal system. These areas of our body are lined with mucous membranes. Of course the allergy can also be introduced by injection (including vaccinations) but this is less common and very hard to prove.

Mucous membranes function as protection, support, nutrient absorption, and secretion of mucus, enzymes, and salts. In the case of allergies the protection role fails.

From a naturopathic point of view it makes sense to help the body restore the protection role of the mucous membranes. Conventional medicine has gone down the path of trying to modify the immune response to the allergen. It seems more logical to us to focus the treatment on restoring the mucous membranes to good health and the body to normal function. After all, the majority of your immune system actually functions out of these mucous membranes and so the restoration process is also restoring good immune function.

The starting point for a naturopathic treatment for allergy is identifying and removing the main causes of the allergy (see section below on how to choose an allergy test). This is usually necessary so that we can remove inflammation from the area affected and start the process of repairing the mucous membranes. There are a number of herbal remedies that have been shown to be effective in this repair process. You will need therapeutic doses of these remedies which are only available from a practitioner qualified in naturopathy, herbal medicine or nutritional medicine.

Once you and your practitioner are satisfied that the repair process is effective, you can then experiment with reintroducing the allergens. At first this should be at very minute doses (as small as a single drop). They should be introduced one at a time with a small increase in the dose every 3 days, so that your tolerance to the allergen builds up slowly and your now healthy mucous membranes have got time to adjust. With more severe allergies it may be necessary to wait around 1 year for the antibodies for the allergen to be fully cleared from your system before introducing the allergen, but in less serious cases it may be possible to start introducing the allergen after a few months of maintaining healthy mucous membranes. Success at this final stage of treatment of reintroducing the allergen can vary greatly between people and will depend largely on the skill of your practitioner. If this process fails, then you will need to continue to avoid the allergen to remain in good health.

## Allergy Tests – How to select between IgE, IgG and ALCAT tests

Based on the knowledge that adverse reactions to foods can be caused by a wide range of factors and involve many parts of the body, it is understandable that diagnostic tests for food reactions may not test all possible causes.

IgE food allergy testing should be used for the assessment of immediate food allergies (generally associated with anaphylactic reactions), whilst IgG food allergy tests analyse delayed food allergies, and ALCAT panels can analyse delayed food allergies as well as reactions to foods that involve histamine release, cytokine release and/or degranulation of leucocytes.

The IgE mediated food allergy is well known, easily diagnosed and usually results in physical symptoms within minutes. The existence and classification of IgG food allergies have been more controversial. The IgG food reactions are difficult to diagnose (without a test) because the time between consumption of the offending food and the physical response may be delayed; even up to 3 days later. The symptoms are also often subtle. In many cases ingestion of the offending food paradoxically masks the symptoms temporarily.

An anaphylactic food reaction is an immediate, severe and often life-threatening reaction to a food. This is mediated by an IgE immune response as set out above.

For the Food IgG Allergy Panels, you must include as many of the foods that are being tested in the two weeks prior to specimen collection. If foods are not included in the diet during this time false negative results may be obtained, as recent exposure to these foods may be required for antibodies to be present in the blood. Foods, however, that have caused an anaphylaxis reaction in the past should never be reintroduced into the diet without the specific guidance of an allergy specialist. For the ALCAT test you do not have to eat any specific foods prior to testing.

The testing lab should advise you about medications that can interfere with the tests. For example for the IgG and IgE allergy tests you usually avoid using anti-histamines, anti-inflammatories and any other immunosuppressive medications for two weeks prior to testing. However, never discontinue prescription medications without first consulting your doctor.

# 9  DON'T BUY IT & WATCH YOUR FINANCES IMPROVE

**Summary**

Decisions throughout the world today are largely driven by money.  At least 2 billion people worldwide have had their health affected by organisations implementing FEAR.  The organisations that put fructose into everything, encourage exercise reduction, continue to use artificial trans fats as a food additive and contribute to a reduction of key nutrients will not change their behaviour unless you stop buying their products.  You only need to look at the poor record that governments around the world have in regard to their slow response to Artificial Trans Fats to know that governments will not act quickly enough to support your return to good health.  However, your purchasing power when combined with just a small percentage of the other 2 billion people affected will have a dramatic effect on the organisations that have implemented FEAR.  These organisations will either need to change to support the FEAR reversal process or they will eventually close down.

The most important financial aspect of FEAR reversal is that as you implement the process you get an immediate boost in energy and enthusiasm. If at the same time you are also implementing the techniques for gaining control of your life then your income will be growing substantially and your total financial position will steadily improve.  We outline in this chapter how most of the actions you can take will reduce your expenses and thus improve your financial situation.

**Now let's look in more detail about this issue and what you can do.**

## Fructose Reduction

The actions you can take in regard to fructose were:

**Strategy 1** – Eat fruit between meals as a snack and never with other food.

**Strategy 2** – Dramatically lower sugar from all sources – this action was for the seriously overweight.

**Strategy 3** – Cut out only major sources of fructose and sucrose – this action was for people trying to lose smaller amounts of weight.

**Strategy 4** – Wean yourself off the sweet taste – this is applicable to everybody.

All of the above save you money by not buying foods and drinks containing fructose and sucrose.

## Exercise

The actions to improve your exercise included

**Strategy 1 – Build exercise into your daily routine**

**Strategy 2 – Replace time watching television with exercise**

**Strategy 3 – Get professional help**

**Strategy 4 – Interval Training**

**Strategy 5 – Check that your routine covers all aspects of exercise**

**Strategy 6 – Exercise your gastrointestinal system**

**Strategy 7 – Gain Control of Your Life**

**Strategy 8 – Find the Reason If You Feel Too Tired To Exercise**

Strategy 3 of getting professional help was only to get advice on how to perform an exercise and so is a one-off expense and should not be very expensive. You don't need to allocate money for expensive gyms or expensive gym equipment. In fact you may be able to raise some money by selling television sets if you have more than one. Walking to some places instead of driving will also be saving money. You may also find that other things that you are implementing are also saving money such as driving to a cheap parking area and walking the rest of the way to your work. You may also find that as electrical equipment around the house needs replacing you are replacing it with cheaper manual equipment.

## Artificial Trans Fats

The strategy here is to avoid any foods containing artificial trans fats. If this is part of an overall reduction in your food intake then you will be saving more money.

## Reduced Key Nutrients

The suggested strategies were

**Strategy 1 – Have a professional review your diet**

**Strategy 2 – Supplement for the obvious deficiencies**

**Strategy 3 – Drink plenty of water**

**Strategy 4 – Include plenty of vegetables in your diet**

**Strategy 5 – Check meal sizes**

Having a professional review your diet is a one-off cost and should not be expensive. There is plenty of competition between supplement suppliers so you should be able to purchase the key ones that you need for relatively low costs. Many people take supplements unnecessarily and this will save you money as you start focusing just on the key ones that you need. Good quality water is available at much lower cost than sweetened drinks, so if you start drinking more water and no sweetened drinks you will be saving significant amounts of money. Vegetable prices can be expensive in some areas but if you shop around you will be able to find good produce at reasonable prices. As demand for fresh vegetables increases, growers will increase capacity replacing crops that were previously grown for the fructose content. Increased capacity by farmers may help keep prices of vegetables low. By checking meal sizes you will generally be consuming less in total quantity than you were previously consuming, so overall there will be a saving in food costs.

## Gaining Control of Your Life

The strategies suggested are

**Strategy 1 – Analyse your own behaviour**

**Strategy 2 – Develop a plan**

**Strategy 3 – Implement Time Management Techniques**

**Strategy 4 - Learn to Listen**

**Strategy 5 - Think Win/Win**

**Strategy 6– Stress Reduction**

**Strategy 7 - Visualisations & Affirmations**

All of these strategies can be implemented without you spending any money. In fact, when you combine these strategies with the FEAR reversal process you find that your outlook becomes positive, you have plenty of energy and plenty of spare time. If you didn't have a job at the start of this process, you will be well on your way to now having one. If you started this process in a poor paying job, you will be well on your way to improving the income you are generating from work.

So the conclusion is clear. By not buying the products or services that have generated FEAR you have substantially improved your financial position. Your purchasing power when combined with the 2 billion other people affected by FEAR will drive changes that smart business people will take advantage of and they will supply effective solutions.

# 10  HOW TO TURN McDONALDS INTO McHEALTHY

To illustrate that large organisations can change to work with FEAR reversal let's look at doing something that most people would regard as impossible. Let's turn your local McDonalds restaurant into a place that supports good health. We will call our rejuvenated restaurant 'McHealthy'.

Remember, FEAR is what we are overcoming so we will do it letter by letter.

**F = Fructose in everything** – so here are some simple actions to overcome this:

• Stop selling sweetened drinks at the food counter – remove them to the cafe or 'drink selling' area and put up a warning sign that says "Sweetened Drinks Should Not Be Consumed With Food As This Could Make You Gain Weight".
• Examine each food item for its fructose content and replace the items with the biggest amount of fructose. So, as an example, all sauces which currently are high in fructose would become fructose free and be replaced with a range of healthy herb and spice sauces. Tomatoes which are high in fructose would be replaced with a fructose free vegetable or alternatively the quantity of tomato in each product could be reduced.

**E = Exercise reduction** – this one is easy to overcome – just install gym equipment in a suitable section of the restaurant away from the food area. Maybe a sign would help that says "Why not take advantage of our exercise equipment before you eat – it will improve your appetite and your health". Free puzzles could be provided at the counter to encourage some mental work out as well. The restaurant could also point out that they are giving your gastrointestinal system a good work out by using whole grain buns and including vegetables with all meals.

**A= Artificial Trans Fats** – some McDonalds restaurants around the world are already tackling this issue and have statements on their websites saying that all their food is completely free of Artificial Trans Fats. It is just a matter of requiring all suppliers to the restaurant to guarantee they have no Artificial Trans Fats in their products.

**R= Reduced Key Nutrient**s – this one is not that hard to overcome either –

• The protein, saturated fat and other key nutrient content of each meal could be specified on each meal pack so you know how much you are getting.
• Some outdoor seating could be provided so that you could eat in the sun and get your vitamin D at the same time.
• Whole grain buns could be used instead of highly refined buns.
• A new McHealthy multivitamin could be sold at the food counter which contains vitamin D3, vitamin K2 and a good balance of the other key vitamins and minerals that we have mentioned.
• Free water coolers could be provided to encourage the drinking of water.

So there you have it, by reversing FEAR you get a new 'McHealthy' restaurant in just four simple steps. And you thought it was impossible!

# 11　A PEOPLE'S HEALTH REVOLUTION

You have probably realised by now that the process of FEAR reversal and returning from a disease state to good health is largely in your hands as an individual. Government organisations have demonstrated their limited ability to act on your behalf. The commercial organisations that are currently inflicting FEAR on consumers will modify their behaviour as you stop buying products that are not healthy. However, none of this means that you are alone in your attempts to get yourself into good health. There are at least 2 billion people in the world today that have been affected by the elements of FEAR. These 2 billion people all have a common goal, they all want to get healthy and be free of disease so that they can make the most of their lives.

We have seen examples throughout the world of how the internet and social networking sites can unite people behind a common cause and make significant changes to their lives. If people can unite to change governments and stop oppression then people can also unite to spread the knowledge about FEAR reversal and getting healthy.

The internet and social network sites allow many of the 2 billion people to find out quickly about FEAR reversal and this means that a 'People's Health Revolution' is possible. Those not connected to the internet can still be advised by family and friends. The starting point for this revolution is to apply the FEAR reversal strategies to yourself and demonstrate by example how well they work. You are then in a position to communicate to other people who know you and trust your opinion. To try to convince a large number of people to change without people setting an example will not work. The 'People's Health Revolution' will only occur if you as an individual, or possibly you as a family group, apply the changes to yourself and then be an example to others.

We encourage you to reverse FEAR, get healthy, tell others about your success and become part of the 'People's Health Revolution'.

# ABOUT THE AUTHORS

Ron Fisher and Caryn Wichmann are both qualified naturopathic doctors and are registered in Australia as naturopaths and nutritionists. They are the founders and principals of the Perpetual Wellbeing Clinic which is a Naturopathic and Nutritional Medicine clinic in the city of Brisbane, Australia.

Their formal qualifications are:
Ron Fisher, N.D, BHSc(Nat), GradDipBus(Acc), ATMS, CPA, FAICD
Caryn Wichmann, N.D, BHSc(Nut), BHSc(Nat), ANTA

While treating clients at the Perpetual Wellbeing Clinic, Ron & Caryn would regularly come across people with complicated health issues that could not be resolved by conventional drug treatment or by traditional natural medicines. They made a decision to devote hours of unpaid research to each one of these cases to find out what was the underlying cause and come up with solutions. The result of this work was creative solutions to health problems and a dramatic improvement in the treatment protocols that were used for all their clients.

Ron & Caryn decided to spread the results of their work more broadly by publishing several books including this book on weight loss and others covering most areas of natural medicine including cancer, gastrointestinal diseases and pregnancy and preconception protocols.

The principles that guide our work, our lives and everything you will find in this book and on our website (www.natmed4u.com) are:

- First do no harm – since Hippocrates all medical practitioners have followed this principle and we know that all those who care about people will also follow this principle,
- Negotiate better outcomes for everyone – although hard work the results are worth the effort,
- Take personal responsibility for your actions,
- Lend a helping hand, and
- Use the best available scientific knowledge to constantly improve your health.